ABC OF ALCOHOL

ABC OF ALCOHOL

edited by
ALEX PATON MD FRCP

with contributions by
KEN O LEWIS, JOHN F POTTER, E BRUCE RITSON,
JOHN B SAUNDERS,
GEOFFREY SMERDON, RICHARD SMITH

Published by the BMJ Publishing Group
Tavistock Square, London WC1H 9JR

First Edition 1982
Second Impression 1984
Second Edition 1988
Second Impression 1989
Third edition 1994
Second Impression 1996
Third Impression 1997
Fourth Impression 1998

British Library Cataloguing in Publication Data

A catalogue record for this book is available from the British Library

ISBN 0-7279-0812-X

Printed in the United Kingdom at the University Press, Cambridge
Typesetting by Apek Typesetters, Nailsea, Bristol

Contents

CONTRIBUTORS

KO LEWIS, MSc, PhD, *principal biochemist, Dudley Road Hospital, Birmingham*

A PATON, MD, FRCP, *retired consultant physician*

JF POTTER, DM, FRCP, *professor of medicine for the elderly, University of Leicester*

EB RITSON, MD, FRCPsych, *consultant psychiatrist, Royal Edinburgh Hospital*

JB SAUNDERS, MD, FRCP, *director, drug and alcohol services, Royal Prince Alfred Hospital, Sydney*

GH SMERDON, MB, FRCGP, *general practitioner, Liskeard, Cornwall*

RSW SMITH, MB, MRCP, *editor, British Medical Journal*

PREFACE TO THE THIRD EDITION

Some people, including doctors, do not believe that alcohol misuse is a medical problem except when there is serious physical harm. Plenty of arguments can be mustered to refute this view. The frequency of alcohol misuse and its many guises touch the lives of all of us. General practitioners are in an ideal position to detect heavy drinking and to give advice because they see so many people; hospital doctors can stop problems developing because ill people are likely to heed their advice. Alcohol misuse provides a rewarding opportunity to practise holistic medicine and to work with other health professionals.

In spite of these and other arguments some doctors are wary of getting involved because of an image of alcohol misusers as time consuming, difficult to manage, manipulative, and, by and large, incurable. In fact this applies to only 6% of those who need help, and the purpose of the *ABC of Alcohol* is to widen horizons so as to provide a core of knowledge that will give practitioners the confidence to deal successfully with the great majority of people who misuse alcohol.

The new edition has been thoroughly revised and, where possible, figures updated, though statistics are still unreliable in the alcohol field. Greater emphasis has been placed on social problems, which far outweigh those caused by physical harm. Twelve years ago, when these articles were first written, experts were predicting an epidemic of alcohol misuse in Britain. Fortunately, levels of consumption have flattened out in the past few years, but this does not mean we should relax our efforts to help those at risk, especially if the targets proposed in *The Health of the Nation* are to be met.

Although the *ABC* is meant as a general introduction for doctors, I hope it will be of some value to other health professionals and social workers, who have much to offer both to those who misuse alcohol and to doctors. I thank them and my fellow contributors, from whom I have learnt a great deal about alcohol misuse, and Barbara Horn and Deborah Reece for their expert editorial assistance.

Alex Paton
July 1993

PREFACE TO THE FIRST EDITION

Alcohol consumption has doubled in Britain in the last 20 years, and at the same time all the measurable forms of alcohol-associated damage have also increased dramatically. The same has happened in most Western countries and in many Third World countries. Few would deny the pleasures of alcohol, and yet it may damage not only individuals but also families and whole communities in different ways. Every health and social worker—indeed, probably every individual—in Britain will be presented with some manifestation of alcohol damage. Yet at the same time as the problems have increased our thinking on alcohol has undergone a revolution.

This book which consists of articles published in the *BMJ* and therefore held up for criticism to 95 000 readers, presents the latest thinking and information on alcohol problems. A full understanding of this multifaceted problem means considering information as diverse as the pharmacological effects of alcohol and the impact of advertising on alcohol consumption. The two parts of this book aim at providing much of what is required. The first part, by Dr Alex Paton and his colleagues, presents in a straightforward and uncomplicated way, with generous use of illustrations, what the non-specialist needs to know about understanding and managing alcohol problems, while Dr Richard Smith's more discursive part surveys current research, thinking, and controversies. Alcohol problems cannot be ignored, and we hope that this book provides an easy way to understanding them.

Stephen Lock
1982

DEFINITIONS

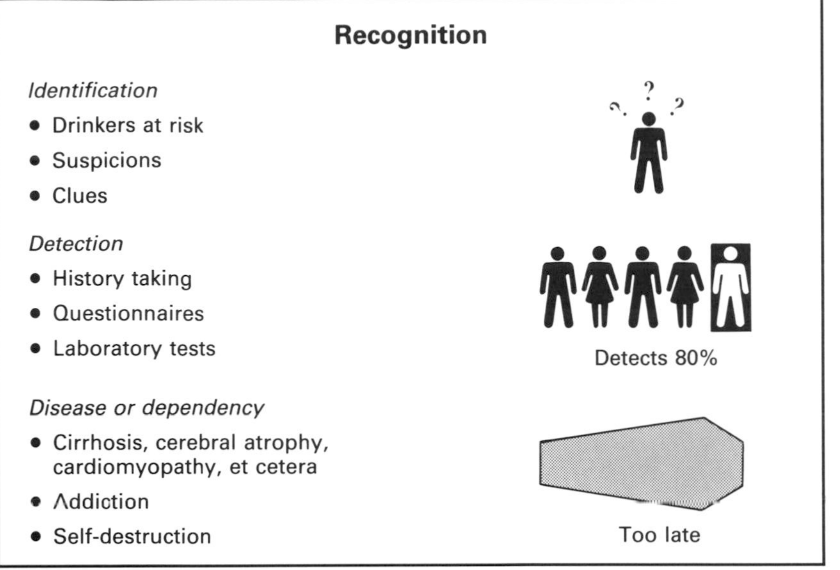

Confused thinking about alcohol misuse arises from *(a)* disagreement over definitions, *(b)* different ways of expressing alcohol consumption, and *(c)* lack of awareness, among doctors and others, of the hazards associated with excessive drinking.

The purpose of these chapters is to provide background information and practical guidelines about alcohol misuse, so that health workers may become more sensitive to an increasingly common social phenomenon and can take action at an early stage, before serious damage has been done.

No single disease

Categories of misuse

Heavy drinking—Either continuous or intermittent (binge) drinking is potentially harmful and therefore important to detect early

Problem drinking—Associated with domestic, occupational, financial, medical and legal problems, which can be overcome by reducing or stopping drinking

Dependence—Implies addiction to alcohol and is commonly irreversible

"Alcoholism" and "alcoholic" are no longer acceptable terms to describe a person's drinking, because they imply a single "disease" and stigmatise the affected individual. It is better to use the term "alcohol misuse" to indicate excessive or repeated consumption that may cause social, psychological, or physical problems, or lead to dependence (addiction). There are many different types of misuse and a wide range of associated problems. The latter are not simply related to the amount of alcohol drunk, because factors such as constitution, sex, social background, occupation, dietary habits, and patterns of drinking contribute to individual susceptibility.

In practice it is helpful to divide misuse into heavy drinking, problem drinking, and dependence.

Range of drinking

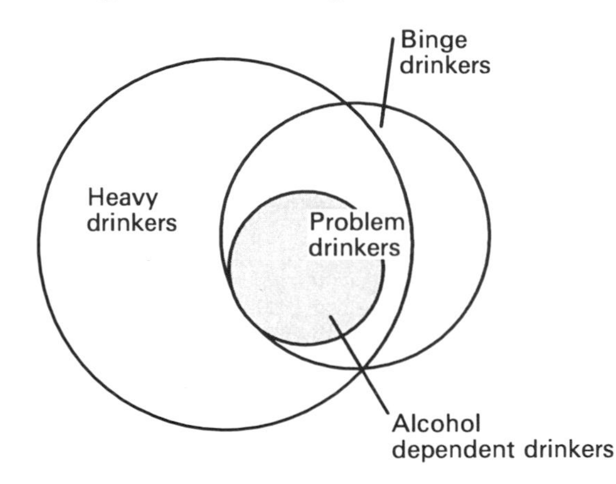

Some examples may make clear the wide range of alcohol misuse. A few particularly sensitive people, women more often than men, harm themselves physically from drinking "social" amounts of alcohol. This may be a true hypersensitivity; if such individuals could be identified, they would be warned to avoid alcohol altogether.

People can damage, and sometimes kill, themselves during a drinking bout. Intoxication alone may cause medical, social, and legal problems.

Heavy drinking, if prolonged, causes serious physical damage, such as cirrhosis, heart disease, and brain damage in a proportion of people who drink heavily, yet it may have no effect on the individual's personal relationships or performance at work until disease supervenes.

Problem drinkers often continue drinking in spite of the physical, psychological, and social problems that their drinking causes.

The *dependent* (addicted) *drinker*, who has an especially high alcohol intake, seems totally unable to stop in spite of the havoc he or she causes, and is at risk of severe withdrawal symptoms without alcohol.

Features of alcohol dependence

- Drinking more than 10 units daily
- Tolerance to alcohol: blood alcohol levels greater than 150 mg/100 ml without drunkenness
- Repeated withdrawal symptoms; morning shakes relieved by alcohol
- Repertoire narrowed by drink
- Compulsion to drink in spite of problems
- Abnormal laboratory tests

These last three categories account for most of the questions addressed in these chapters.

"Skid row" drinkers may have repeated convictions for drunkenness but in general do not develop physical disease, perhaps because of periods of enforced abstinence. *Binge drinkers*, on the other hand, seem as liable to physical problems as regular heavy drinkers. Some people who drink to excess may be a nuisance to themselves or others because of personality problems or compulsive tendencies, without necessarily becoming dependent on alcohol or developing physical disease.

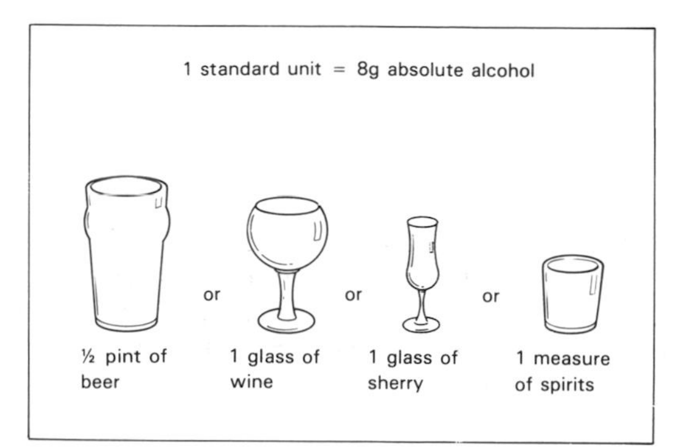

Epidemiological comparisons of alcohol misuse are bedevilled by lack of uniformity in designating quantities. Statements such as "five drinks a day" are meaningless, if, for example, quantity and type of alcohol are to be related to physical damage. Measurement of alcohol intake in terms of grams (g) of absolute alcohol daily is gradually being adopted for scientific and professional use. Quantities can be quickly calculated by a nomogram (see below).

One pint of beer may vary in alcohol content from 12 to 40 g according to strength; one glass of wine, one small glass of sherry, or one "single" of spirits can be considered for purposes of calculation to contain 8 g (they vary from 7 to 11 g).

An agreed measure that can be readily understood by lay persons is also needed. The "standard unit" used in Britain is one centilitre (again about 8 g) of absolute alcohol, equivalent to half a pint of average-strength beer, a glass of wine, a small glass of sherry, or a "single" of spirits.

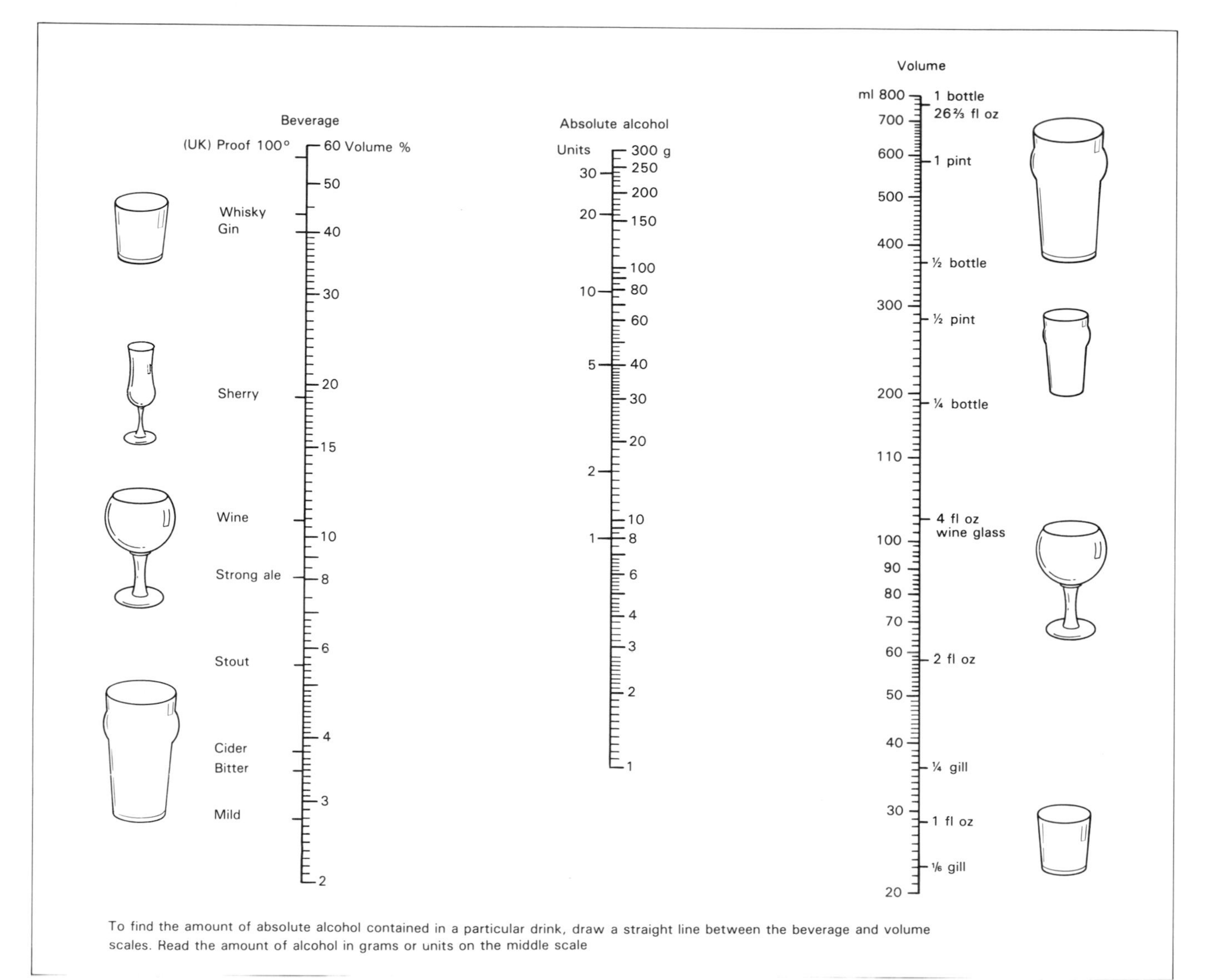

To find the amount of absolute alcohol contained in a particular drink, draw a straight line between the beverage and volume scales. Read the amount of alcohol in grams or units on the middle scale

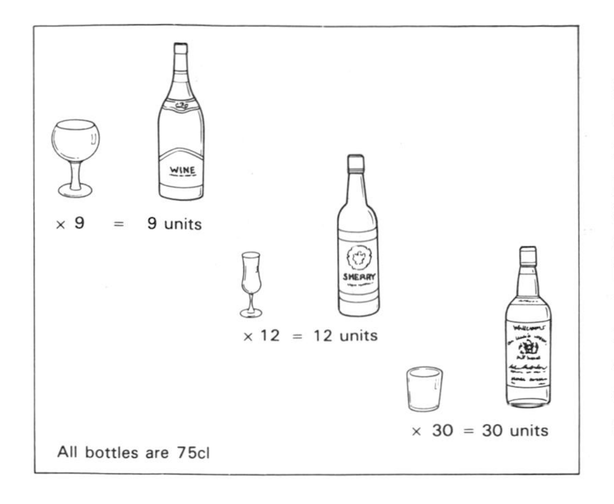

An arbitrary level for the development of cirrhosis has been given as six pints of beer, a third of a bottle of spirits, or half a bottle of sherry daily (60–80 g alcohol ($7\frac{1}{2}$–10 units)), but this may be too high in some individuals. Thresholds of 120–160 g (15–20 units), once proposed for physical damage, are certainly excessive, and there may be no absolutely safe limits. In France, for example, thresholds as low as 60 g ($7\frac{1}{2}$ units) alcohol daily for men and 20 g ($2\frac{1}{2}$ units) for women have been suggested for liver damage. Men who drink more than 56 g (7 units) alcohol a day and women who drink more than 40 g (5 units) may be defined as heavy drinkers. Only the individual who is teetotal is entirely free from risk, though there is epidemiological evidence that alcohol intakes of 1–2 units daily may protect against coronary heart disease; light use of alcohol may reflect a healthier lifestyle.

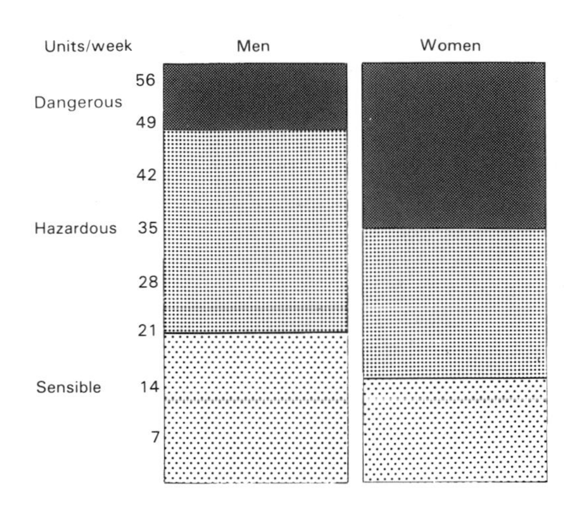

There may be no truly safe daily level of consumption. The Scottish Health Education Coordinating Committee has therefore suggested a "norm of 2–3 pints 2–3 times a week" (or equivalent), and the Health Education Council up to 21 units a week for men and 14 units for women, with occasional days of abstinence. These "sensible limits" have been endorsed by the Royal Colleges of Physicans, Psychiatrists, and General Practitioners.

In the present state of knowledge women who wish to conceive are advised to abstain completely; after the first trimester an occasional drink is permissible.

NATURE OF THE PROBLEM

Statistics on alcohol misuse are unreliable

Estimates of the number of people who misuse alcohol are unsatisfactory because of lack of agreement over definitions, difficulties in establishing harmful levels of intake, and problems with carrying out the necessary surveys. One survey of drinking habits, for example, uncovered less than half the consumption known from sales of alcohol.

Drinking patterns vary according to race, religion, class, and geographical region. In Britain more money is spent on alcohol than on any other commodity. About 10% of people are teetotal; of those who drink, three-quarters come to no harm.

Numbers

	Adult population 43 million	*General practice* 2000
Drinking above sensible limits	7.3 million	340
Heavy drinkers	4 million	186
Problem drinkers	800 000	37
Dependent drinkers	400 000	19

Presently one in four men and one in ten women are believed to be drinking over sensible limits of 21 and 14 units a week respectively. With a population of 43 million between the ages of 15 and 75 (WHO 1992) almost equally divided between men and women, this would mean about 5 million men and 2.3 million women "misusing" alcohol.

Distribution of drinkers

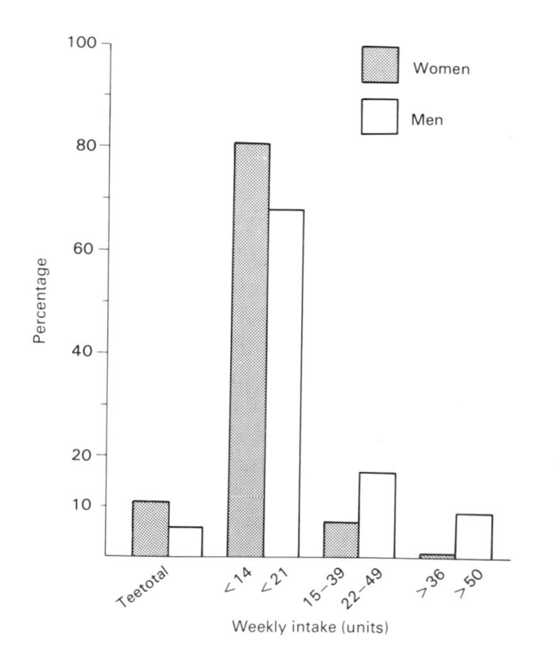

The number of habitual heavy drinkers is estimated at about 4 million, of whom about one-fifth are problem drinkers and one-tenth are alcohol dependent. Relatively few in the alcohol dependent group conform to the unemployed, dispossessed stereotype of the "skid row" drinker conspicuous in larger cities. For every problem and dependent drinker several members of the family suffer from the effects of his or her drinking.

A general practitioner with 2000 adult patients would be expected to have about 186 heavy drinkers, of whom 37 are likely to be having problems and 19 to be dependent on alcohol. Previous surveys suggested that only one in ten heavy drinkers was known in a practice. By asking questions about drinking the general practitioner has an opportunity to detect alcohol misuse at a stage when it is treatable, and to provide more accurate data about the distribution of drinking among the population.

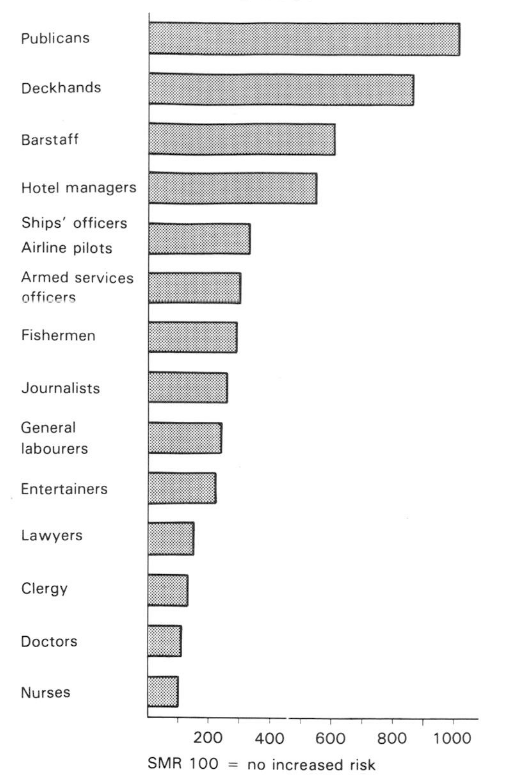

Alcohol misuse is a multifactorial condition; different people misuse alcohol for different reasons, and it is misleading to lump everyone together. Unfortunately, attempts at classification have not yet been successful. Early twin and adoption studies suggested that inheritance was a powerful cause, but Robin Murray and his colleagues calculate the strength of the genetic component at about 36%, compared with 46% for intrafamilial but not genetic influences, and 18% for purely environmental factors. Up to 50% of dependent drinkers have a family history of alcohol misuse; they tend to start drinking young and rapidly become addicted, and exhibit other types of deviant behaviour.

The majority of misuse results from a mixture of constitutional and environmental factors. The former include low self-esteem, habit, boredom, loneliness, lack of interests and skills, anxiety and depression (though true depression is uncommon) and ethnicity. Examples of environmental factors are availability, peer pressure (especially when young), a competitive lifestyle, occupation, unemployment, difficulty in adapting to an urban or alien environment, and a reaction to acute stress such as a bereavement.

Certain occupations, such as those in which individuals are subject to stress or where alcohol is easily available, are associated with high levels of drinking. Perhaps in some cases individuals are attracted to certain occupations by an unexpressed need to work where alcohol is readily to hand and acceptable. Publicans and others in the catering trade, seamen, members of the armed services, and airline pilots are among those whose death rates from cirrhosis are 3–10 times the standardised mortality ratio (SMR). Alcohol misuse is a problem among professionals, including doctors, though there has been an encouraging fall in SMR among doctors from 300 to 110 in the past few years.

Patterns of drinking

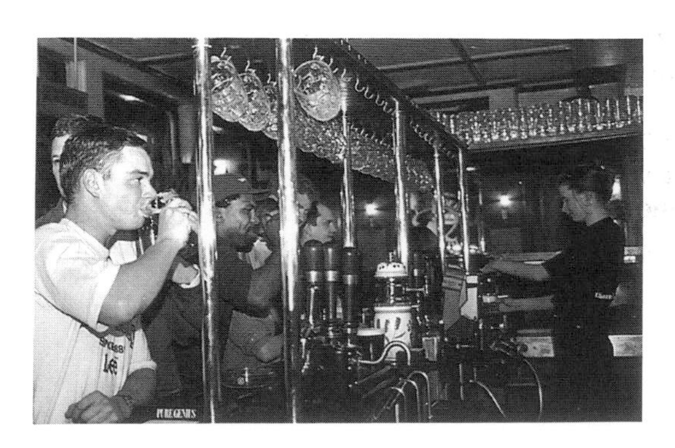

Beer accounts for two-thirds of the alcohol drunk in Britain, though its share of the market is declining as wine and spirit drinking increase, especially among women. Similar trends are reported in other industrialised countries.

While the legal age for drinking is 18, the average age at which drinking starts has fallen from around 16–18 to 10–11 since the early 1970s in both boys and girls. One in eight children between the ages of 7 and 15 claims to drink regularly, and about 13 000 children under 16 drink in pubs. The earlier drinking begins, the more likely are heavy consumption and alcohol-related problems in later life.

The most striking change has been the rise in drinking in women, especially among professionals, 10% of whom drink over sensible limits compared with 5% of unskilled women. Alcohol-related problems have also increased. Twenty years ago deaths from alcoholic cirrhosis were five times as common in men as in women; the ratio is now 1·5:1. Nearly as many women as men seek help from counselling services; problems, especially physical damage, arise at an earlier age and after a shorter period of drinking.

The highest rates of drinking occur in the 18–24 year age group: 36% of men and 17% of women drink above sensible limits. Most will subsequently reduce their intake, but serious harm can be caused at this time by intoxication and even from physical damage and dependence.

Alcohol misuse among elderly people seems to be commoner than suspected; one estimate, thought to be conservative, is that 13% of the population over the age of 60 are heavy drinkers. Alcohol misuse may add to their proneness to physical illness as well as to falls and confusion.

Recognition

- Many heavy and problem drinkers do not seek help because they do not admit that their drinking is harmful
- Many people are harmed by somebody else's drinking but are reluctant to seek help for fear of offending the drinker
- Serious physical damage and dependence are frequently irreversible
- Doctors should concentrate on detecting heavy and problem drinkers, for whom advice and information about sensible drinking—"minimal intervention"—is likely not only to be successful but to cost little in time, resources, and money

Up to one in five healthy men attending health screening programmes have biochemical evidence of heavy alcohol consumption; they are a selected population. About 25% of patients in hospital are found to be heavy drinkers. Figures are likely to be high in medical wards because of the number and variety of medical problems related to alcohol, and in accident and emergency and orthopaedic departments because of trauma. Psychiatric admissions associated with alcohol misuse total 17 000 annually; with increasing emphasis on outpatient management, the true figure in psychiatric patients is probably much higher. No specialty is immune, and all patients attending hospital should be questioned about their use of alcohol. Many hospital doctors fail to recognise heavy drinkers and even problem drinkers. Greater awareness is needed so that patients can be offered treatment at a time when they are likely to be receptive, and to provide better information on the true extent of the problem in hospital and its cost to society.

WIDER ISSUES

Changes in alcohol consumption over the centuries (England)

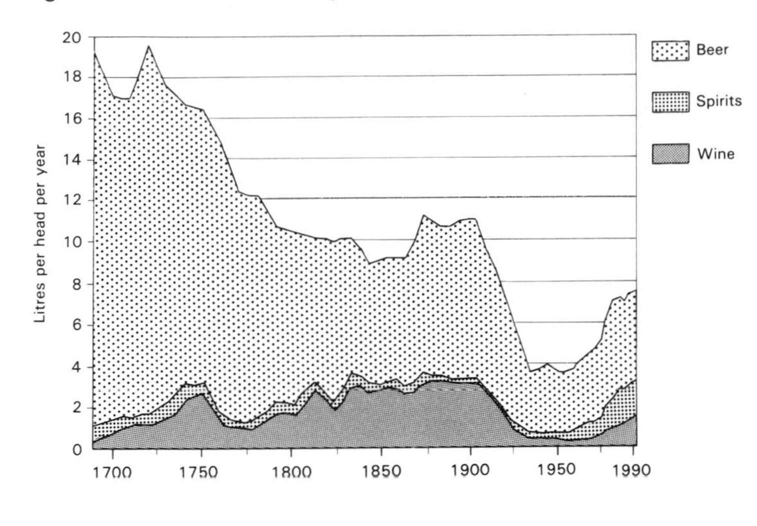

While doctors are primarily concerned with the physical problems of alcohol misuse they must not lose sight of the much more frequent social consequences of excessive drinking. Health and social workers need to have some knowledge of the social, economic, and political issues associated with use of alcohol.

For much of this century Britain has been one of the most abstemious countries in the Western world. A steady rise in alcohol consumption accompanied by a dramatic increase in indices of harm—death rates from cirrhosis rose sixfold—began in the 1960s. By the early 1980s consumption per head of population (over the age of 15) had doubled from 5 to over 9 litres a year. Figures began levelling out towards the end of the decade and now stand at just under 8 litres. Similar trends have been noted in other European countries, where per capita consumption is a good deal higher than in Britain.

Ledermann hypothesis

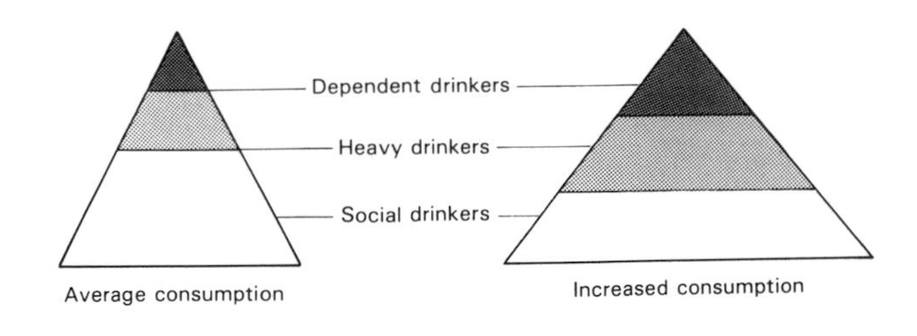

The French demographer S Ledermann demonstrated that changes in shape of the distribution curve of per capita consumption of alcohol could be used to predict the amount of harm that would result. Rises and falls in consumption are accompanied by upward and downward trends respectively in indices of harm. An increase of X in consumption will usually produce an increase in damage closer to X^2 than to X.

Ledermann curve

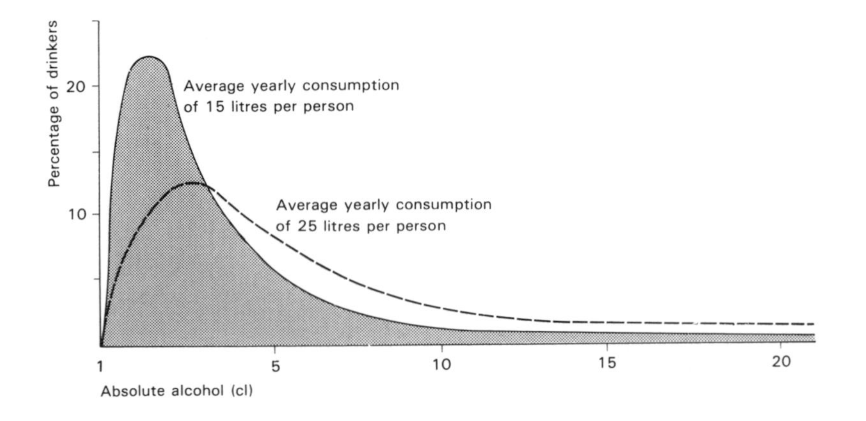

The Ledermann curve has a continuous (log normal) distribution rather like that for blood pressure; there is no sign of separate populations of "alcoholics" and "normal drinkers." A rough rule is that 10% of the drinking population consumes half the total amount of alcohol drunk. A rise in consumption is likely to increase disproportionately the number of heavy and dependent drinkers; anything that reduced consumption would have the greatest effect on social and heavy drinkers because of their numbers. The Ledermann hypothesis has been disputed but it can provide an approximation of the numbers of people in a given population drinking different quantities of alcohol.

Social harm

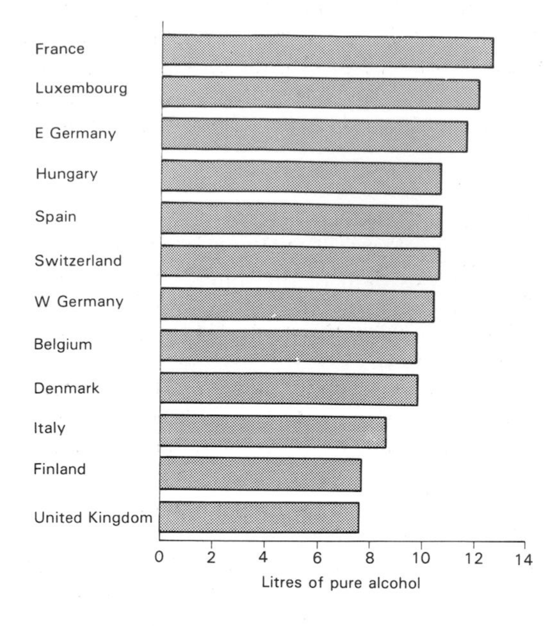

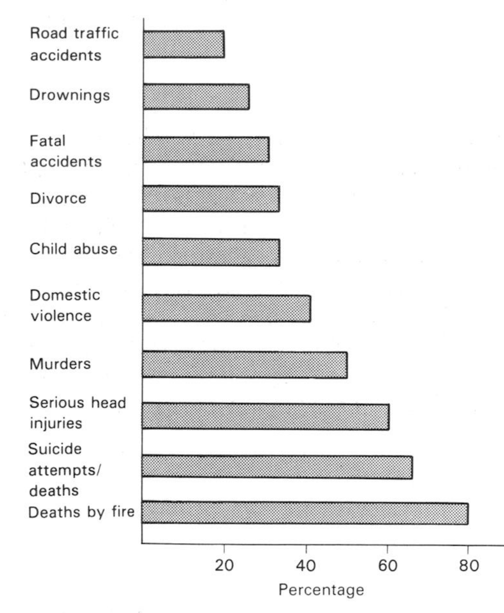

Alcohol plays a part in many aspects of social harm, but it is not necessarily the sole or even the most important factor. Families of people who misuse alcohol may suffer as much as, or even more than, the individuals themselves. A third of problem drinkers give marital discord as one of their concerns; a third of divorce petitions cite alcohol as a factor. As long ago as 1975 a survey of wife battering found that half the husbands were "frequently drunk," and episodes of heavy drinking were present in a further fifth.

Conflict between parents is likely to affect children. They may be the recipients of violence or sexual abuse; 20–30% of cases are quoted as being associated with alcohol misuse. Neglect is more common, and children may be affected by poverty resulting from parental drinking. Children from such families attend child guidance clinics ten times as often as their peers. Nevertheless some children exhibit remarkable resilience and ability to cope.

Alcohol misuse is found in a significant proportion of the homeless, in whom unemployment, loss of family, financial difficulties caused by drinking, and psychiatric illness contribute to a degrading existence.

Violence and accidents are closely associated with alcohol misuse in Western societies such as Europe, Scandinavia, and North America. A peak of nearly 190 000 convictions and cautions for drunkenness in England and Wales occurred in 1980, when per capita consumption was at its highest. Some reduction in consumption and changes in police policies have been associated with a decline to around 130 000. Intoxication is a common cause of violence, especially among the young, but the popular view that drinking is solely responsible for the behaviour of "lager louts" and football hooligans may be too simplistic. Incidents of violence associated with alcohol are increasingly reported in patients attending accident and emergency departments.

Homicide is commonly associated with drinking in both the perpetrator and victim. Two-thirds of offenders serving prison sentences for burglary admitted drinking before carrying out a crime. Alcohol misuse is common among all types of prisoner: 40% of women in Holloway for failing to pay a fine were thought to be misusing alcohol.

Convictions for drink-driving reached a peak of over 66 000 in 1980; they have since declined by 40%. The number of accidents on the roads related to alcohol has fallen by 60%: in 1991 there were 800 deaths (about a fifth of the total), 4010 serious injuries, and 13 960 slight injuries. These encouraging results are thought to be due to campaigns against drink-driving and improvements in road safety. The only figure that has shown a rise is the number of accidents among pedestrians who have been drinking.

Alcohol is responsible for a substantial number of deaths from accidents in the home and at work, from fire and by drowning.

Morbidity and mortality

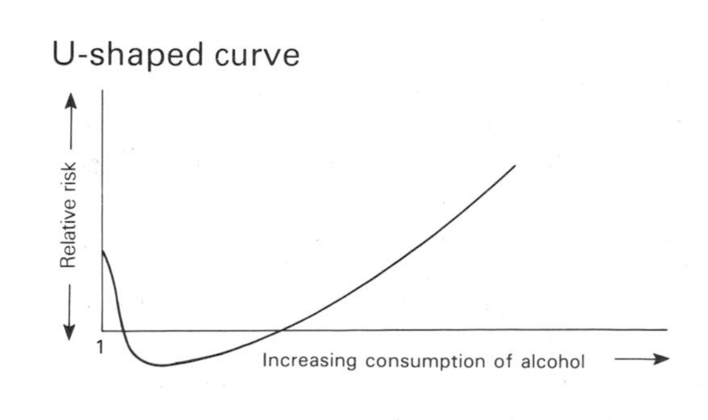

In some conditions, such as hypertension, liver cirrhosis, and cancers, there is a dose response relationship between alcohol use and morbidity—the greater the amount drunk, the more the harm done. An interesting variation of this association is the U-shaped curve, in which the relative risk of death is greater than one in those who do not drink at all and in the heaviest drinkers, but is lower than one in moderate drinkers. This suggests a "protective" effect of alcohol in moderate drinkers, especially for coronary heart disease. The exact significance of this finding is at present uncertain, and while drinking within sensible limits may protect against coronary heart disease, any benefit from larger amounts is likely to be offset by the considerable risk of damage from other causes.

Annual death rates from cirrhosis are used as an indicator of mortality from alcohol misuse. Figures in Britain are thought to be too low by a factor of as much as five, partly because of failure to diagnose

Alcohol misuse can harm minds, bodies, families, societies, and economies

the condition and from reluctance of doctors to certify alcohol as a cause of death. Other causes include cancer, especially of the aerodigestive tract, sudden death and some types of heart disease, and the result of intoxication and dependence, drug overdose, and suicide.

Current estimates of the total number of deaths range from 25 000 to 40 000 a year; these are based on indirect evidence rather than counting the number of deaths actually attributed to alcohol misuse. Whatever the true figure, the important point is that many deaths are premature: 500 under the age of 25, for example, and around 200 000 life years lost.

Cost equation

Credit		*Debit*	
	billions		*millions*
Revenue: excise duty	£5·5	Absenteeism	£780
exports	£1·5	Unemployment	£180
Employment 125 000 jobs		Offences	£40
		Traffic accidents	£112
		Health services	£120
		Premature death	£704

Costs to society of alcohol misuse are incurred through lost productivity, material damage, and responses to associated medical, social, and legal problems. Industry, for example, loses £770 million and 14 million days through sickness absence. Alan Maynard and his colleagues produced a total figure of nearly £2 billion in 1989, based on losses to industry, costs of health care, support for problem drinkers and their families, and the expense of accidents and crime. It is impossible to assess pain and suffering or the financial burden on individuals and families.

Against these figures must be set the revenue obtained by government from duty and exports—currently £7 billion (£13 000 a minute)—and the 125 000 people employed in the drinks industry.

- The range of alcohol problems is too great to be solved by health and social workers alone
- A "treatment response" can have only limited success because many people do not seek help
- Many alcohol problems are not easily treated
- Public education on its own can do little
- Political action can reduce alcohol misuse

Public education alone has had little effect on alcohol misuse. Programmes fail because of naïve expectations, insufficient attention to the level of public knowledge, lack of involvement of those targetted, and inadequate resources. The Heath Education Authority's alcohol budget is only £4 million. Mass-media campaigns, especially on television, are expensive, but they can raise questions and start debates, which can be taken up at local level. Small campaigns, "owned" by the people, are likely to be more effective: they can be tailored to suit the audience, checks can be made on understanding, questions answered, anxieties allayed, and courses of action suggested. Messages need to be constantly reinforced.

Political action

Price, consumption and cirrhosis death rates

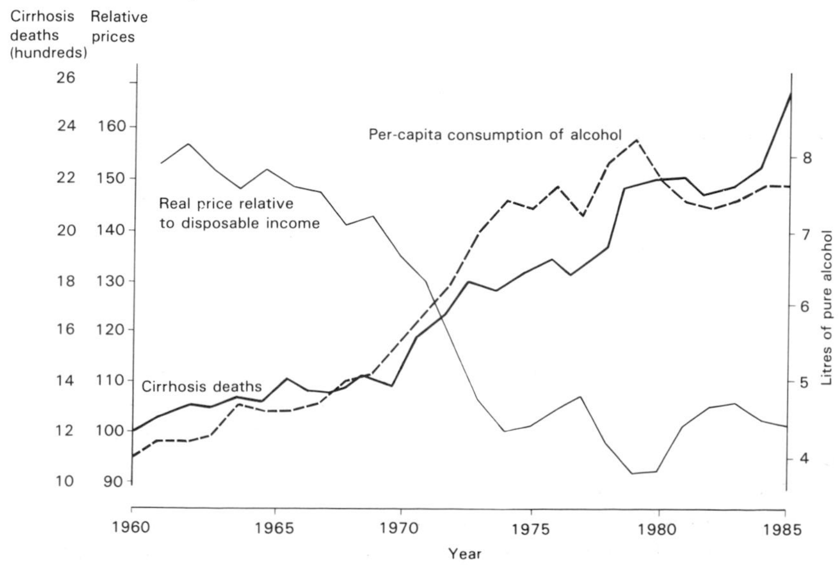

In the end political action is necessary because the most effective regulator of alcohol consumption is price. Consumption is higher in countries in which alcohol is inexpensive than in those in which it is dear. Rises and falls in price and consumption have mirrored each other for the past three centuries in Britain. Between 1960 and 1980 the gap between price and affordability narrowed, so that the price of a drink fell to a third of its cost in the 1930s, and consumption rose sharply. In Scotland a price rise in the 1981 budget was followed by an 18% drop in consumption and a 16% fall in 14 possible ill effects of drinking. Proposed harmonisation of alcohol taxes throughout the European Community (which would reduce the price of some drinks in Britain by a third) would be expected to increase consumption.

Alcohol consumption, drunkenness offences, and deaths from alcoholism and cirrhosis, England and Wales 1860–1978

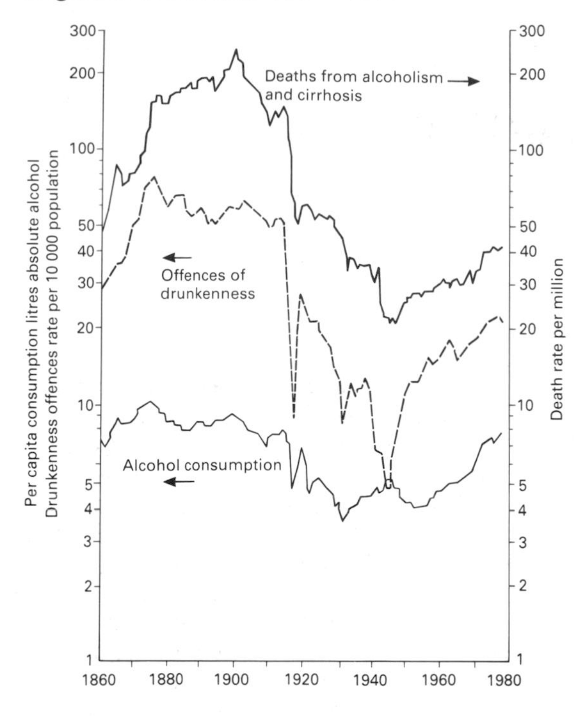

Another way to influence drinking is to alter availability, either through outlets like off licences and supermarkets or by changing licensing laws. When buying alcohol is easy, as in Britain, such changes probably make little difference; there is no evidence of increased drinking since the licensing laws were liberalised in 1989. The virtual abolition of restrictions on the amount of alcohol that can be brought into the country duty-free may have the opposite effect.

Although consumption in Britain is low compared with that in many other European countries, the harm done by excessive drinking cannot be ignored.

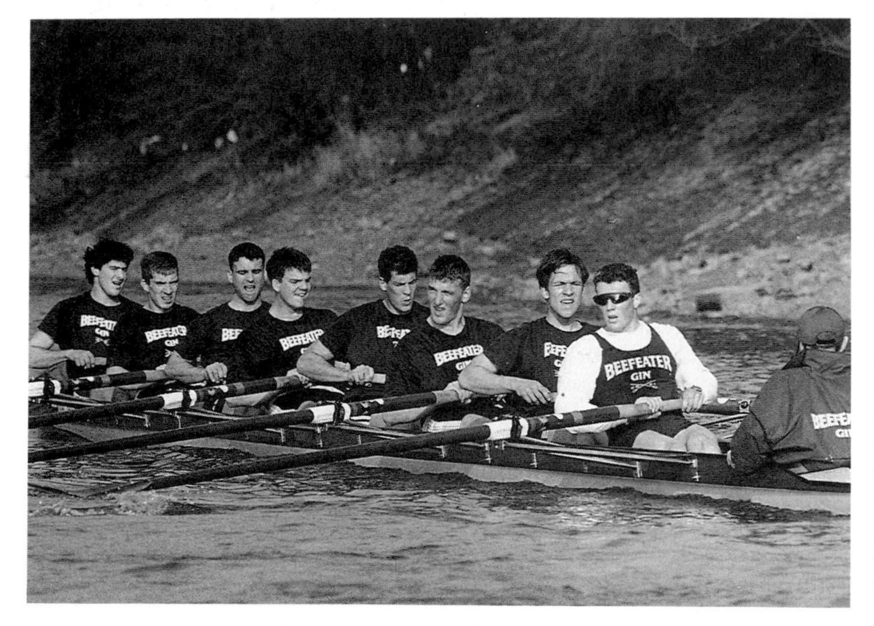

The drinks industry spends £300 million on advertising and sponsorship, and this is widely believed to increase consumption. The industry responds that promotion merely persuades people to drink one brand rather than another. Countries that have restricted advertising have reported reductions in drinking especially among the young—a special target for the industry. Children and adolescents obtain information about alcohol from television advertisements, where reference to alcohol occurs on average every 6·5 minutes. Even if this does not encourage drinking, it will influence personal preference and patterns of use. The industry accepts a code of practice in which alcohol advertising should not be associated with glamour, sex, youth (people drinking should be at least 25), and sport, yet in practice the guidelines are frequently broken.

Weight of public opinion might eventually influence government action. Eighty per cent of people in this country would like to see tighter controls on underage drinking and drink-driving (only one in 250 drivers is currently detected), random breath tests (which have reduced driving accidents by 35% in New South Wales), restricted advertising, and labelling of alcoholic drinks. So far the government has turned down these suggestions.

ALCOHOL IN THE BODY

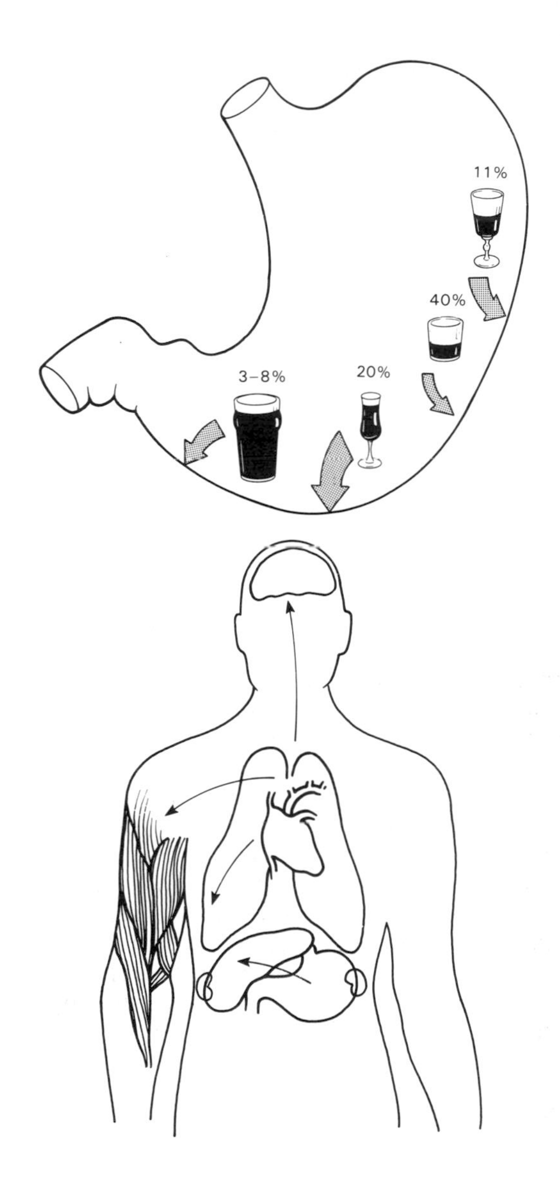

Alcohol is a drug, and it is important that doctors know something of its handling by the body and some of its physiological effects.

Alcohol is absorbed from both stomach and small intestine, but is more rapidly absorbed from the latter. The rate of absorption is variable: it is most rapid when alcohol is taken on an empty stomach and when the concentration of alcohol in the drink is between 20% and 30%. Thus sherry or vermouth (about 20% alcohol) raise blood concentrations more rapidly than beer (3–8%), while spirits (40%) delay gastric emptying and are absorbed best when diluted. Food, and particularly carbohydrates, retards absorption considerably: blood concentrations may not reach a quarter of those in the fasted state.

Alcohol is distributed throughout the body water, so most tissues—heart, brain, and muscles—are exposed to the same concentrations as in blood. Concentrations are higher in the liver, which receives blood via the portal vein from stomach and small bowel. Little alcohol enters fat because of its poor blood supply, so that women, with more subcutaneous fat and a smaller blood volume, achieve higher blood and tissue concentrations than men, even when the amount of alcohol is adjusted for body weight. A further factor may be that women have lower levels than men of alcohol dehydrogenase in the stomach, so that less alcohol is metabolised before being absorbed.

Blood alcohol concentrations vary according to sex, size, and body build, previous exposure to alcohol, type of drink, whether it is taken with food, and whether drugs that affect gastric emptying are used. Initial blood concentrations are particularly high in patients who have had a partial gastrectomy.

Alcohol is eliminated predominantly by hepatic metabolism; only 2–5% is excreted unchanged in urine or breath. About one unit is eliminated per hour. The amount customarily taken by heavy drinkers represents an enormous metabolic load, and the liver's capacity for dealing with such quantities is relatively limited, although the heavy drinker may adapt by enzyme induction for a considerable time before the liver finally fails. Half a bottle of spirits, for example, is equivalent in molar terms to 500 g of aspirin or 1·2 kg of tetracycline.

Acetaldehyde

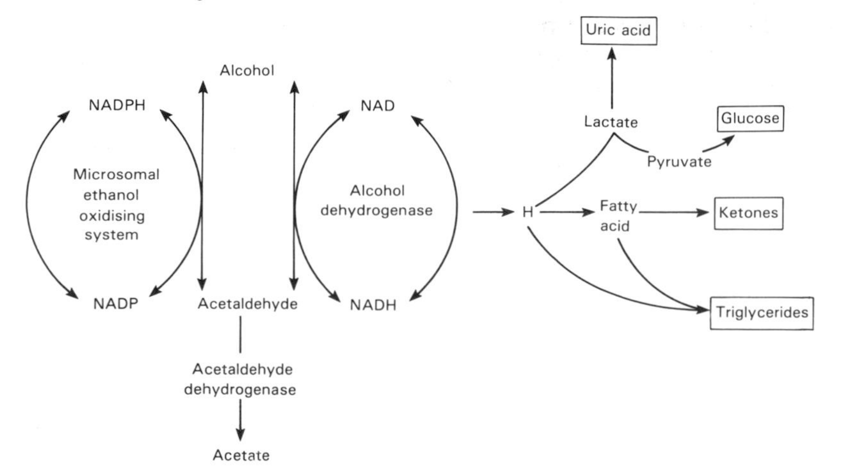

Most alcohol is metabolised to acetaldehyde, a highly reactive and toxic substance, which has been suspected for many years of being responsible for the physical damage caused by excessive alcohol consumption. Attempts to incriminate it have so far been unsuccessful. It is normally rapidly metabolised to acetate, which is not toxic, and concentrations in most tissues are extremely low.

Several metabolic abnormalities result from the oxidation of excess alcohol, including over production of lactic and keto acids, retention of uric acid, hyperlipidaemia, and accumulation of fat in the liver.

Peak concentrations and rate of removal

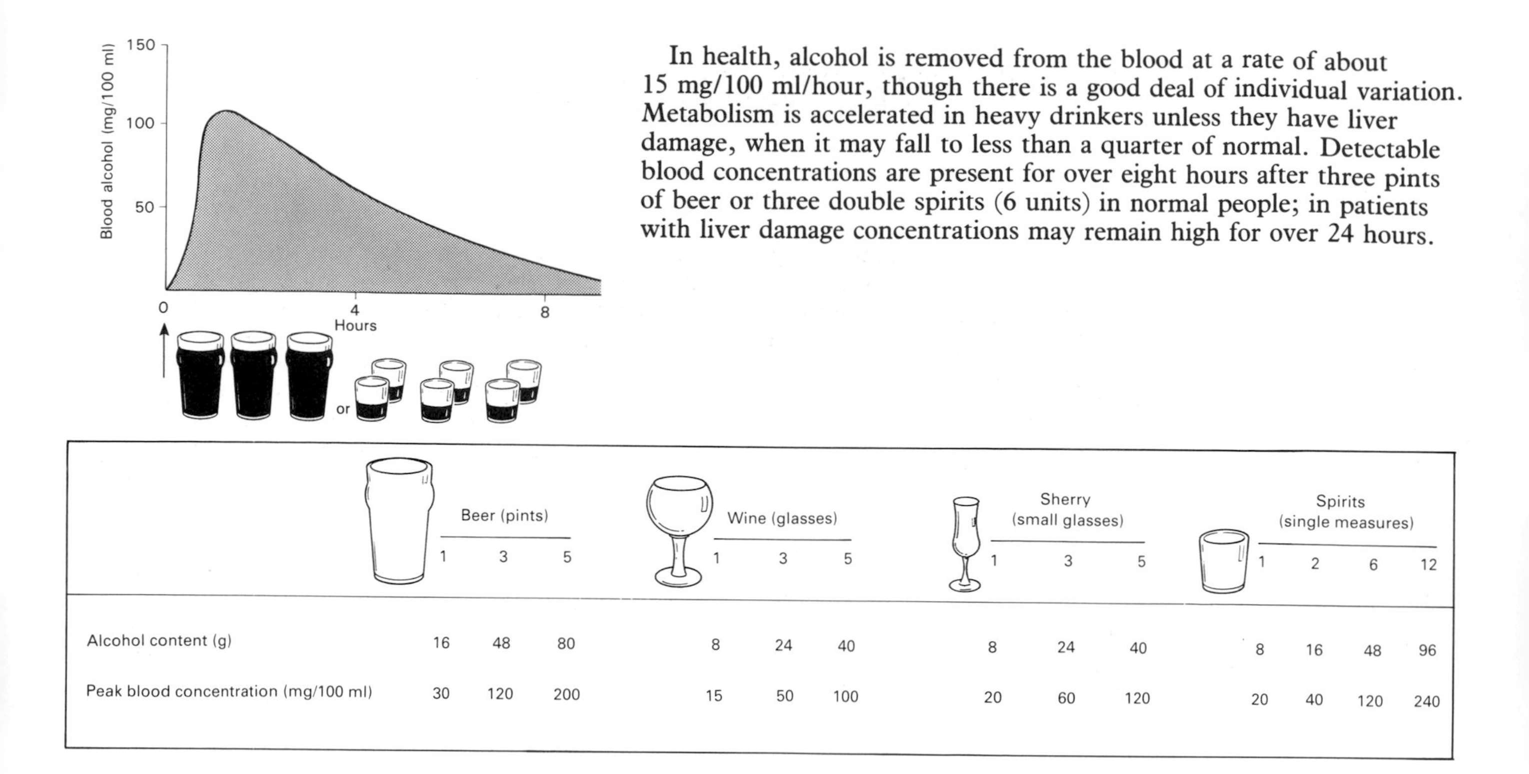

	Beer (pints)			Wine (glasses)			Sherry (small glasses)			Spirits (single measures)			
	1	3	5	1	3	5	1	3	5	1	2	6	12
Alcohol content (g)	16	48	80	8	24	40	8	24	40	8	16	48	96
Peak blood concentration (mg/100 ml)	30	120	200	15	50	100	20	60	120	20	40	120	240

In health, alcohol is removed from the blood at a rate of about 15 mg/100 ml/hour, though there is a good deal of individual variation. Metabolism is accelerated in heavy drinkers unless they have liver damage, when it may fall to less than a quarter of normal. Detectable blood concentrations are present for over eight hours after three pints of beer or three double spirits (6 units) in normal people; in patients with liver damage concentrations may remain high for over 24 hours.

Effect on behaviour

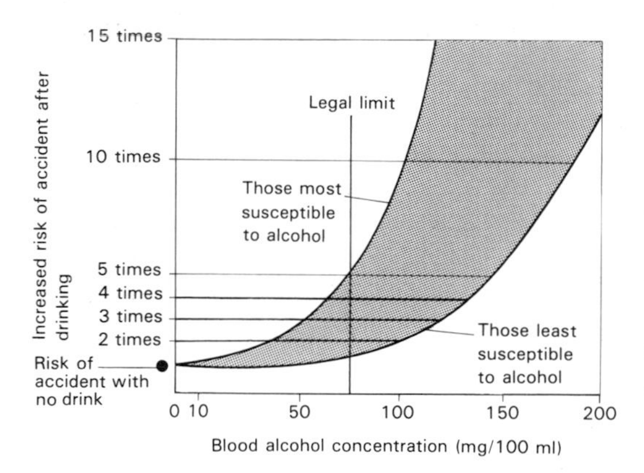

Alcohol has a euphoriant and disinhibiting effect, but even at low blood concentrations (around 30 mg/100 ml (6·5 mmol/l)) the risk of accidental injury increases. In a simulated driving test bus drivers with blood alcohol concentrations of 50 mg/100 ml (10·9 mmol/l) thought they could drive through obstacles that were too narrow for their vehicles. At 80 mg/100 ml (7·4 mmol/l) the risk of a road accident is more than doubled; at 160 mg/100 ml (34·7 mmol/l) it increases more than tenfold. Dysarthria and ataxia occur at concentrations of 160–200 mg/100 ml (43·4 mmol/l), when loss of consciousness may result. Concentrations above 400 mg/100 ml (86·8 mmol/l) are commonly fatal, especially if a sedative drug is also taken.

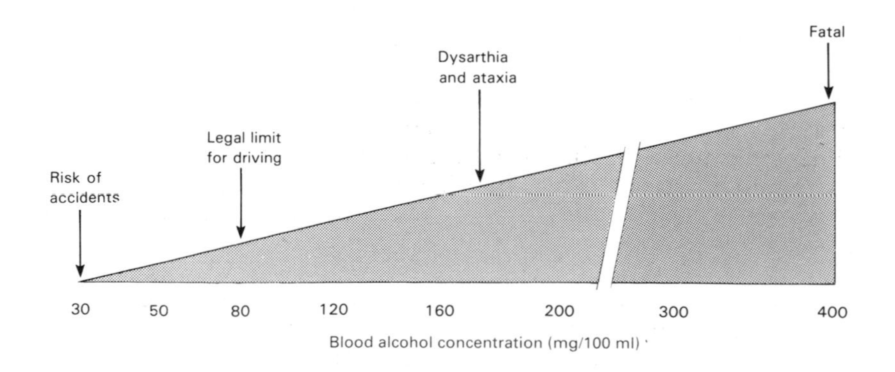

ASKING THE RIGHT QUESTIONS

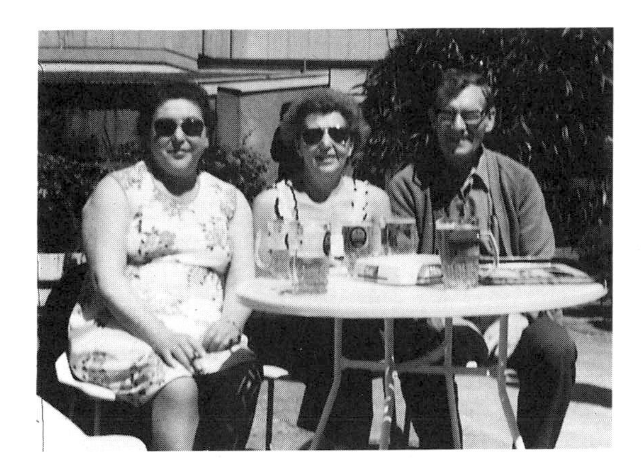

Many people who are not concerned with alcohol misuse believe that it is impossible to get reliable information about drinking patterns. The reasons given are *(a)* self-deception and guilt on the part of the drinker; *(b)* the difficulty in many cases of heavy drinkers—for example, barstaff—being able to assess their intake; and *(c)* failure of doctors to take an adequate drinking history. Even so, 80% of those who drink to excess give a drinking history that tallies with that from other sources, and if quantities are accepted as approximations, valuable information can be obtained. It is the part played by alcohol in an individual's life that is important.

During history taking questions about alcohol consumption should always be included (and recorded), both in hospital and in general practice. It is important that they be asked in the same neutral manner as other questions. They may be included with questions on symptoms or past illnesses that are relevant to the diagnosis or combined with questions on lifestyle, such as smoking, diet, exercise, and self-medication.

A positive response will allow the doctor to explore the pattern of drinking in greater detail. He or she can make a reasonably accurate assessment by asking what the patient has drunk in the previous week. If the answer is nothing, the patient is unlikely to be misusing alcohol. If drinking is denied, the question should be asked why: abstention may be due to religious or temperance reasons or because of former misuse.

- Do you smoke? What do you smoke? How much?
- How long have you been smoking?
- Do you drink? What do you drink?
- Roughly how much?
- How long have you been drinking?
- Do you take tablets or medicines? What are they for?

If heavy drinking is suspected and the patient seems evasive, one technique is to use a facetious approach and to set the figure very high—for example with beer, "Thirty pints a day?"—and gradually to reduce the quantities asked. The astute observer can usually gauge the approximate level by the subject's reaction. Do not be misled by individuals who say they used to drink heavily but do not do so now. Do not ask a patient whether he or she is an alcoholic; the question will almost certainly be resented because of the implied stigma, which conflicts with the individual's self-image.

Computers

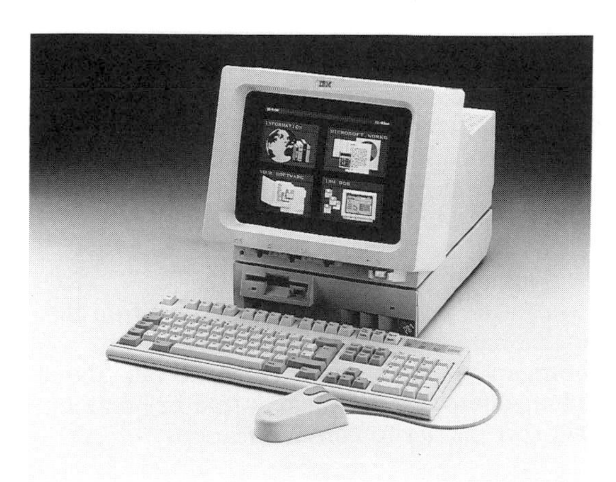

A new refinement has come with the advent of personal computers. Programmes consisting of a series of questions on drinking habits, quantities consumed, and problems associated with heavy drinking have now been designed. They can be stored on floppy discs and used with several commercial computers. This approach has been successful in obtaining reproducible histories from patients with a wide range of educational backgrounds and intelligence.

For screening patients in hospital or general practice it is appropriate to establish the pattern of drinking and average daily alcohol consumption. "Quantity-frequency" questionnaires can be used as an aide memoire; self-administered versions are particularly useful when time is at a premium. They can also be given to the spouse. Questions are asked about the type of alcohol taken; for each type, the frequency of drinking, using fixed choice categories; the usual quantity on each drinking day; and the maximum amount on any one occasion. The average daily consumption can then be calculated in units of alcohol.

A simpler method is to use a drinking diary in which the patient is asked to note down every alcoholic drink he or she has taken in the previous seven days. This gives a reasonable approximation to intake as established by quantity-frequency questionnaires or by interview.

Questionnaires

Brief MAST

	Circle correct answer	
Do you feel you are a normal drinker?	YES	NO (2 pts)
Do friends or relatives think you are a normal drinker?	YES	NO (2 pts)
Have you ever attended a meeting of Alcoholics Anonymous?.	YES (5 pts)	NO
Have you ever lost friends or girlfriends or boyfriends because of drinking?.	YES (2 pts)	NO
Have you ever got into trouble at work because of drinking?	YES (2 pts)	NO
Have you ever neglected your obligations, your family, or your work for two or more days in a row because you were drinking?	YES (2 pts)	NO
Have you ever had delirium tremens (DTs), severe shaking, heard voices or seen things that were not there after heavy drinking? . .	YES (5 pts)	NO
Have you ever gone to anyone for help about your drinking?	YES (5 pts)	NO
Have you ever been in a hospital because of drinking?	YES (5 pts)	NO
Have you ever been arrested for drunken driving or driving after drinking?	YES (2 pts)	NO
Total score		

Questionnaire for patient attending hospital or GP

Do you drink alcohol . . . . YES NO

If NO, did you ever drink? . . . . YES NO

How old were you when you started? (Age in years)

How often do/did you drink (*Circle*)
Daily/2–3 times a week/Once a week
Weekends only/Once a month/Less

What do you drink? (*Circle more than one if necessary*)

Beer—specify type (mild, bitter, lager, stout, etc).

Spirits/Sherry/Wine/Cider

Other—specify type (home brew, tonic wine, etc).

How much do you drink?

Specify pints of beer

measures of spirits or part of bottle

glasses of sherry, wine, cider or part of bottle

Used you to drink more than this regularly? . . . . . YES NO

Have you ever deliberately cut down on your drinking?. YES NO

Cage

Have you ever felt you ought to *cut* down on your drinking?

Have people *annoyed* you by criticising your drinking?

Have you every felt bad or *guilty* about your drinking?

Have you ever had a drink first thing in the morning to steady your nerves or get rid of a hangover? (*"eye-opener"*)

Several questionnaires have been developed for the diagnosis of alcohol misuse. The Michigan Alcoholism Screening Test (MAST) and the "cage" questionnaire have withstood the test of time. The MAST is available in two versions: the original 25-item questionnaire, which is administered by an interviewer, and a shorter, self-administered version comprising the 10 items of greatest discriminatory value. A score of five points or more on the Brief MAST is taken as diagnostic of alcohol misuse.

Both versions have been used successfully to identify alcohol misuse among general and psychiatric hospital patients. They are useful in screening programmes and for research, but in the clinical setting the shorter "cage" questionnaire, which consists of four items, is more appropriate. Two or more positive replies are said to identify problem drinkers. Neither test should be regarded as more than 75% accurate.

Alcohol questionnaires have the disadvantage that they depend on honest replies from an individual who may be unwilling to admit to social problems or police convictions. They lack the inherent subtlety of the medical interview, and the self-administered versions depend on the patient being well enough and sufficiently motivated to complete them. By concentrating on social problems and symptoms of alcohol dependence they tend to encourage a narrow concept of alcohol misuse. Patients with physical diseases caused by alcohol may never have suffered any of the social consequences of heavy drinking nor have been dependent on alcohol. Indeed, their drinking habits may have been regarded as socially quite acceptable, so that such patients will be missed by this type of questionnaire.

In routine practice there is no substitute for dispassionate face-to-face discussion. Both doctors and patients are reluctant to talk about alcohol; doctors should take a lead in breaking down this barrier to communication.

TOOLS OF DETECTION

Alcohol concentrations

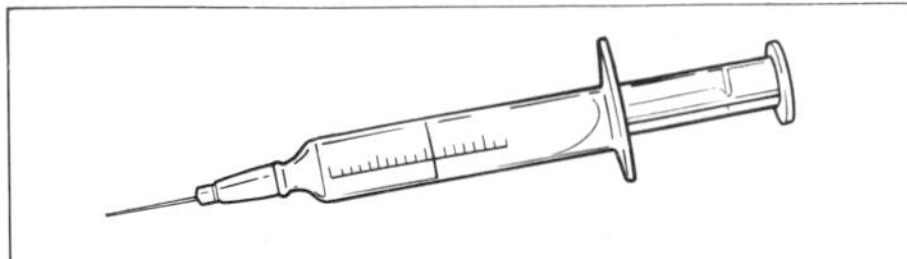

When taking blood samples do not clean the skin beforehand with methylated spirits

The blood alcohol concentration is not used enough as a test for alcohol misuse. It can be measured in toxicology laboratories and in many chemical pathology departments, or, if necessary, in a regional laboratory. Raised concentrations can provide incontrovertible evidence of excessive drinking, and because alcohol is eliminated relatively slowly from the blood appreciable amounts may be found for 24 hours after a drinking session.

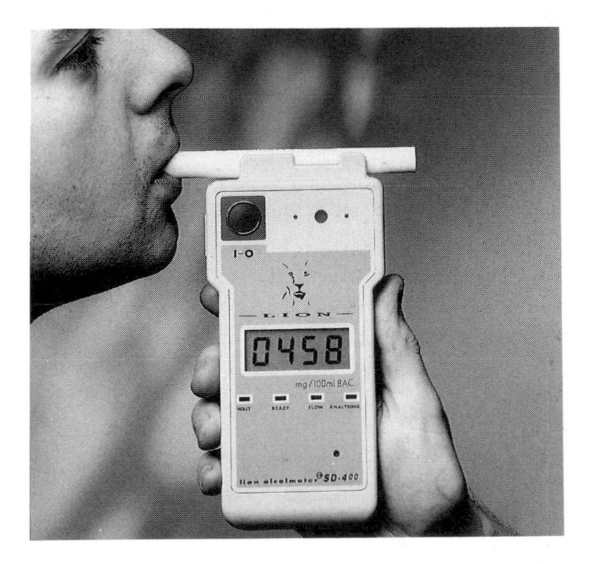

A blood alcohol concentration exceeding 80 mg/100 ml (17·4 mmol/l) (the legal limit for driving in Britain) is highly suggestive of alcohol misuse, especially in the morning, and values above 150 mg/100 ml (32·5 mmol/l) are diagnostic. Such values do not distinguish an isolated drinking bout from chronic alcohol misuse, but if there are no signs of inebriation at concentrations of 80 mg/100 ml (17·4 mmol/l) or more the individual may be assumed to be a heavy drinker. A blood alcohol estimation should always be considered in the unconscious patient: values usually exceed 300 mg/100 ml (65·1 mmol/l) if alcohol alone is responsible.

Breath alcohol measurements reflect blood concentrations, are simple to perform, and provide an immediate result. The Lion Alcolmeter costs £440 and can be used with a minimum of instruction.

Concentrations of alcohol per 100 ml

Blood	*Breath*	*Urine*
50 mg	22 μg	67 mg
80 mg	**35 μg**	**107 mg**
150 mg	66 μg	200 mg
250 mg	110 μg	333 mg

The urinary alcohol concentration can also be measured: a value exceeding 120 mg/100 ml (26·0 mmol/l) is suggestive and one over 200 mg/100 ml (43·4 mmol/l) is diagnostic of alcohol misuse. The sample should be refrigerated and preferably frozen until analysis, otherwise false positive results will be obtained, especially in diabetic patients, because of fermentation of glucose.

Conventional tests: no unequivocal values

	Normal values
γglutamyltransferase (γGT)	< 40 IU/l
Mean corpuscular volume (MCV)	80–90 fl
Urate	120–360 μmol/l
Triglycerides (fasting)	0·85–2 mmol/l
Aspartate aminotransferase	< 25 IU/l
Creatine phosphokinase (CPK)	<150 IU/l

None of the conventional laboratory tests, either alone or in combination, can give an unequivocal indication of alcohol misuse. Those that are highly sensitive are not invariably abnormal. They are affected by other diseases, in particular of the liver, blood, heart, and kidneys, and by drugs, especially those that induce enzymes, such as barbiturates, anticonvulsants, and steroid hormones. Nevertheless, if these causes can be excluded, abnormal values should alert the doctor to the possibility of alcohol misuse before there is physical damage and suggest that advice should be given about reducing alcohol intake or abstaining altogether.

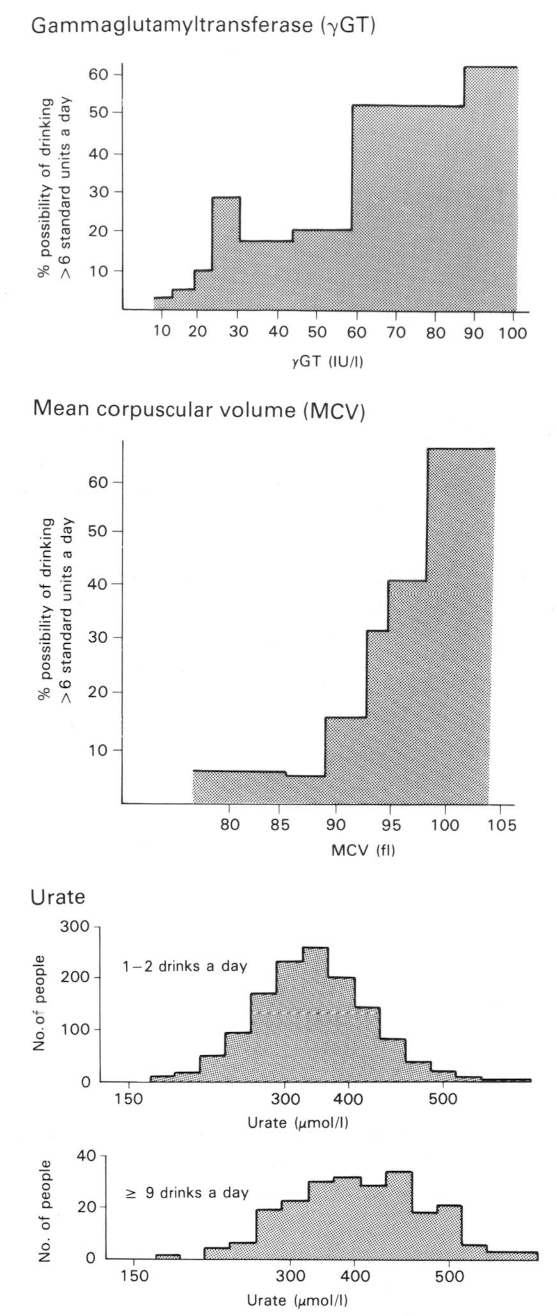

The most sensitive markers of alcohol misuse are the serum concentration of the enzyme γglutamyltransferase (γGT) and the red cell mean corpuscular volume (MCV). Together they will identify three out of four heavy drinkers. Supportive evidence may be obtained from measuring serum urate, fasting triglycerides, and the enzymes aspartate or alanine aminotransferase and creatine phosphokinase.

Measurement of γglutamyltransferase activity is the best screening test available. Values above 40 IU/l are found in about 80% of problem drinkers, both men and women, but do not indicate serious liver damage unless levels are in the hundreds.

A mean corpuscular volume of more than 92 fl is found in about 60% of alcohol misusers and is more commonly raised in women than men. If other causes have been excluded a raised mean corpuscular volume is especially meaningful, since the action of alcohol on the maturation of red cells differs from its effect on biochemical processes in the liver.

Urate concentrations (raised in about half of all heavy drinkers) and fasting triglycerides may be usefully included in a screening profile in men, but they are poor discriminators of heavy drinking in women. A grossly lipaemic serum will sometimes indicate alcohol misuse. Urea concentrations are often reduced because alcohol inhibits enzymes in the urea cycle.

Raised aminotransferase activities indicate liver damage rather than alcohol misuse, being present in over 95% of patients with alcoholic hepatitis and in half of those with fatty liver or cirrhosis.

Creatine phosphokinase activity is raised in nearly half of all excessive drinkers; high values may result from bruising. Because it is not an index of liver function it provides a means of separating detection of alcohol misuse from detection of liver damage.

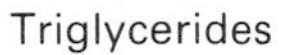

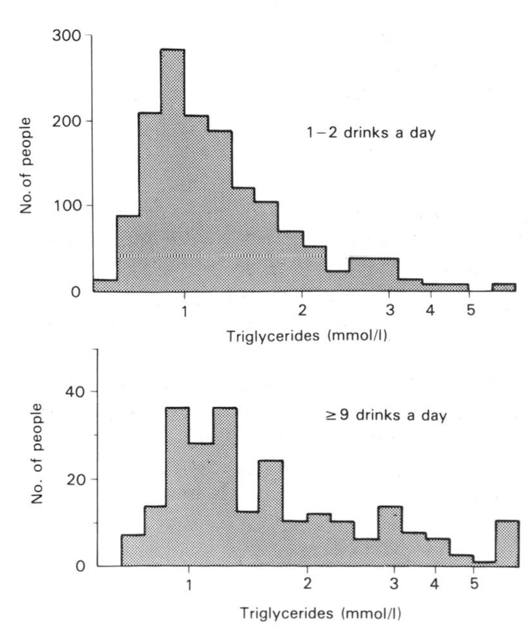

Combined use of γglutamyltransferase and mean corpuscular volume testing provides a simple way of detecting excessive alcohol intake in routine practice. Increasing concentrations of each marker can be directly related to increasing alcohol intake, but they give only a statistical probability that a subject is misusing alcohol. Nevertheless, as their normal distribution is heavily skewed (most results being at the lower end), values in the upper range of normal should be viewed with suspicion if one marker—for example, mean corpuscular volume—is definitely abnormal.

Biochemical markers such as γglutamyltransferase activity return rapidly to normal with abstention from alcohol and may be misleading if measured 48 hours after the last drink. A subsequent rise of 50% or more is strong evidence of resumption of heavy drinking. The mean corpuscular volume, on the other hand, takes up to three months to return to normal after abstinence, reflecting red cell turnover by the bone marrow.

DETECTION IN HOSPITAL

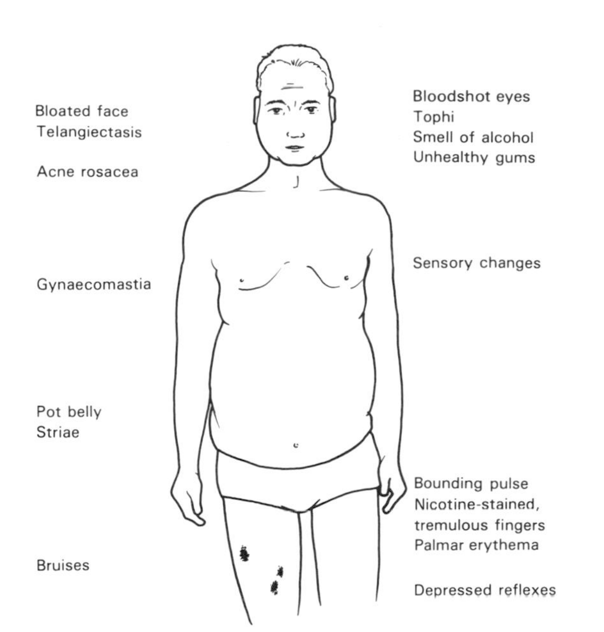

Alcohol misuse has replaced syphilis as the great mimic of disease. Its protean symptoms are compounded by the reluctance of many patients, relatives, and doctors to accept that there is a problem. In addition, the medical approach is that of the doctor looking for gross signs of disease of the liver, heart, brain, or other organs. To concentrate on these is deceptive and unhelpful. By the time they are present the disease is frequently irreversible, and their absence gives a false sense of security.

A few people are referred to hospital about their drinking habits; and a few, who may or may not be known to misuse alcohol, are referred because of hepatomegaly or abnormal liver function tests. These are the minority. Most people who turn out to be problem drinkers have non-specific symptoms which are often vague, multiple, and do not fit readily into any diagnostic pattern; sometimes they may be bizarre. Gastrointestinal symptoms, chest and abdominal pain, and neuropsychiatric disturbances are the most common, but any system may be affected.

Spotting the problem drinker

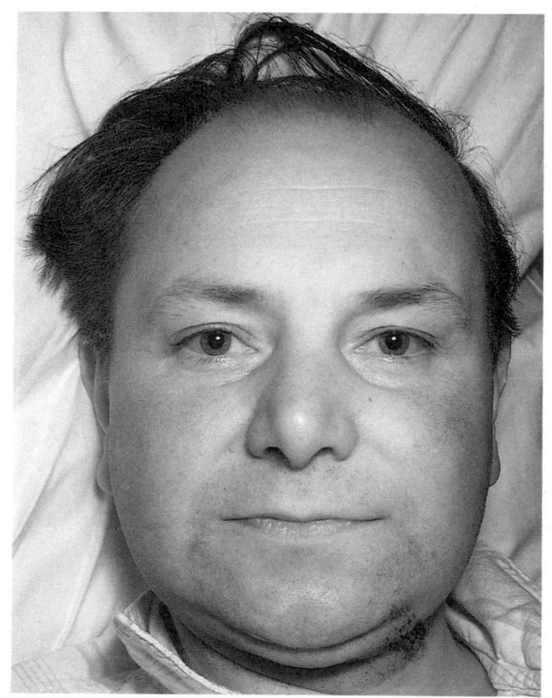

A heavy drinker's history

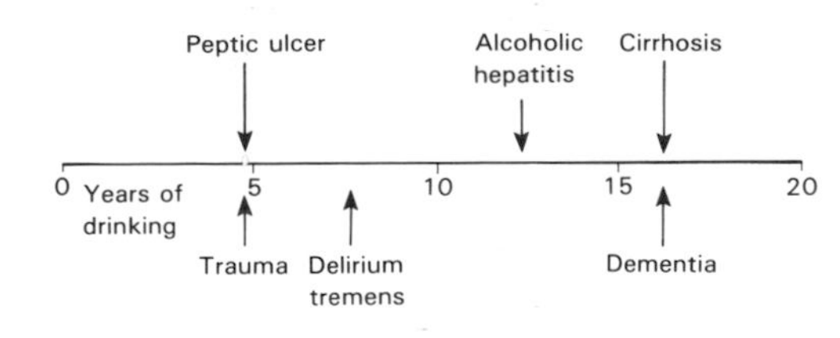

Problem drinkers may be spotted by their brash, jocular, overfamiliar manner, inappropriate to the circumstances of a medical consultation. They may give shifty answers to preliminary questions—denial is almost universal—and it is important not to reveal any suspicions and lose their confidence. Symptoms should be regarded sympathetically and not brushed aside; they will often provide further clues.

Certain features in the history should also raise suspicions: absenteeism from work, especially on Mondays; frequent attendances for unexplained and atypical dyspepsia or for minor gatrointestinal bleeding; hospital admissions for accidents of all kinds or "head injury"; fits, "turns", falls, and neuritis (peripheral neuropathy).

Familial risk factors include alcohol misuse; teetotalism; depression, especially among women; a broken home; and being last in a large family. Drinking by the spouse, drug taking, and heavy cigarette smoking are often associated.

Ethnic origins and religious affiliations should be considered. People of Irish and Scottish descent seem to drink more than the English and to be more prone to physical damage. Other Europeans may have a high prevalence of alcohol problems because they are socially accustomed to high levels of drinking. Jews may drink but intoxication is frowned on. Muslims are, strictly speaking, forbidden by their religion to drink alcohol, but taboos are breaking down, especially among men. Heavy drinking occurs in Asian, Afro-Carribean and other ethnic groups in Britain, but individuals are often deterred from seeking help. More work is needed on the patterns of drinking operating in these communities.

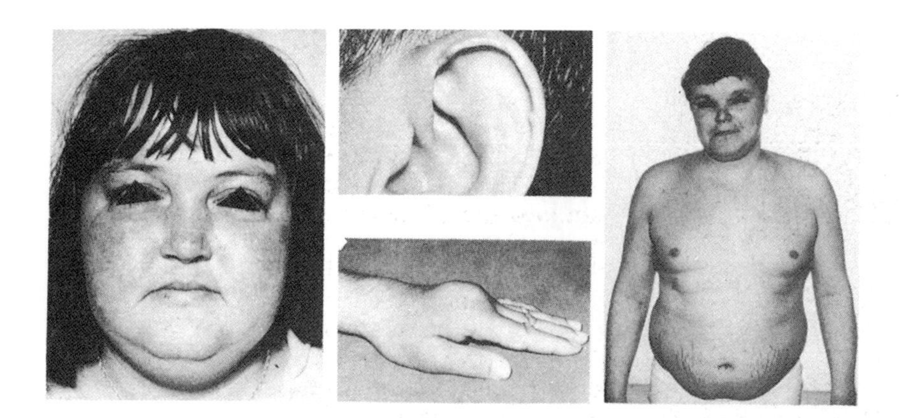

Complaints	Mistaken for	Due to
Gastrointestinal Poor appetite Indigestion Heartburn Vomiting Diarrhoea Bleeding Jaundice	Peptic ulcer Viral hepatitis Gall stones	Oesophagitis Gastritis Enteritis Mallory Weiss syndrome Pancreatitis Alcoholic hepatitis/cirrhosis
Neuropsychiatric Trembling Sweating Insomnia Headaches Blackouts Fits Confusion Inability to concentrate Anxiety or depression Burning legs Coma	Neurasthenia Anxiety state Epilepsy	Withdrawal symptoms Hypoglycaemia Depression Stroke Acute psychosis Encephalopathy Neuromyopathy Dementia Alcohol/drug overdose Subdural haematoma
Cardiorespiratory Palpitations Chest pain Bronchitis "Asthma" Pneumonia	Ischaemic heart disease Essential hypertension	Arrhythmias Hypertension Cardiomyopathy Upper lobe pneumonia Tuberculosis
Infections, including AIDS		Defective immunity
Musculoskeletal Backache Rheumatism Gout Repeated injuries	Idiopathic gout Accidents	Gout Osteoporosis
Skin Bruises/scars Flushing Rashes		Accidents Acne rosacea Psoriasis
Hormonal and metabolic Obesity "Sugar" Breast swelling Reduced libido Infertility	Cushing's syndrome Diabetes mellitus Breast tumour Phaeochromocytoma Carcinoid	Hormonal imbalance
Obstetric and gynaecological Menstrual disturbances Premenstrual tension Delayed fetal growth Stillbirths Congenital abnormalities		Hormonal imbalance? Fetal alcohol syndrome

Signs

Certain signs may be helpful, if present: the bloated, plethoric face, with or without telangiectases or spider naevi; bloodshot conjunctivae; acne rosacea; smell of stale alcohol sometimes disguised by peppermint or heavy aftershave lotion; and raw, red gums which may bleed readily. Facial appearances resembling those of Cushing's syndrome are seen in about a third of patients.

The skin is warm and moist with a fast, bounding pulse, and marked tremor of nicotine-stained fingers (a pseudothyrotoxic state). Other signs, such as palmar erythema, bilateral Dupuytren's contractures, parotid swelling (rare), and gouty tophi, should be sought. Obesity, with a pot belly, gynaecomastia, and striae, are common. Bruising and scarring indicate recurrent falls and brawls.

Clues

The physical consequences of alcohol misuse are well known and this is not the place to discuss them. Successful medical intervention depends on diagnosis before irreversible damage has occurred, and the index of suspicion should be high that alcohol contributes to or causes the following:

Repeated attendance or admissions for relatively minor complaints which cannot be clearly labelled

Fits for the first time in middle age

Gout, whatever the immediate precipitating cause

Mild diabetic symptoms or glycosuria in the young or middle-aged

"Essential" hypertension in men; failure to control the blood pressure with multiple drugs

Atypical cardiac symptoms, arrhythmias or cardiac failure in middle-aged men

Attacks of confusion, especially in strange surroundings or after stress (illness, operation, bereavement, et cetera) and in the elderly

Drug overdoses

Gastrointestinal symptoms where a cause cannot be established

Hepatomegaly, for which no other cause can be found

Anaemia, especially if folate deficient

Lobar pneumonia, especially when it affects the right upper lobe; atypical pneumonias

Atypical endocrine features mimicking Cushing's disease, thyrotoxicosis, phaeochromocytoma, and carcinoid

"Turns" and falls in the elderly

Action

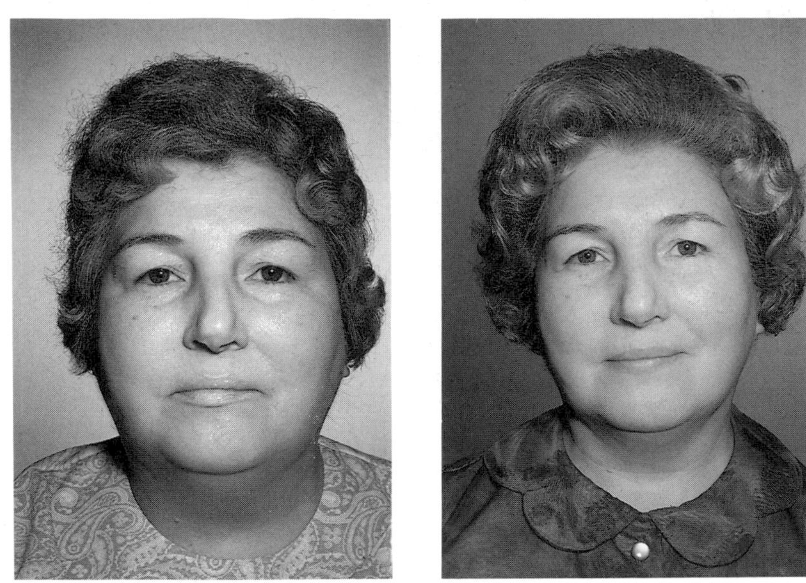

Before (*left*) and after (*right*) stopping drinking.

Patients found to be regularly drinking over sensible limits on history-taking and those who have clinical features suggesting problem drinking should be given advice about cutting down while in hospital, since counselling at this time is likely to be heeded. If necessary, these patients can be provided with one of the many booklets about alcohol misuse, like *That's the Limit*, and referred to the local alcohol agency. The practice of discharging patients after detoxification or treatment for other alcohol-related illness without follow-up is bad medicine; they should always be referred to the local agency or to a specialist clinic. A directory of alcohol services for England and Wales is published by Alcohol Concern.

DETECTION IN GENERAL PRACTICE

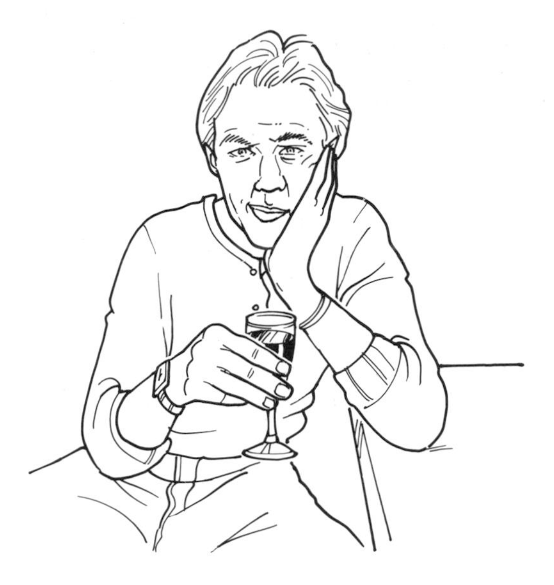

General practitioners, used to dealing with sick individuals, are finding the requirements to examine their patients as a whole population a confusing exercise in changing regulations and numerical manipulations. All patients accepting a new-registration medical check must now be asked about their alcohol intake. All practices are also required, if their Family Health Service Authority (FHSA) so directs, to state in their annual report the number of patients to whom they have given advice about alcohol consumption.

Practices claiming health promotion payment have to report the number of patients (aged 15–74 in six age bands and by sex) whose alcohol consumption is recorded; the number who state that they are drinking amounts exceeding the recommended sensible limits; and the number with this risk factor offered advice, follow up, and health promotion interventions during the year. The targets for these recordings increase from 20% in March 1994 to 75% in March 1998.

These requirements are difficult to meet without computerisation: Read Codes list a range of six consumption levels, but a more helpful classification, which takes account of the different susceptibilities of men and women, is offered by the Royal College of General Practitioners (RCGP).

Who is affected?

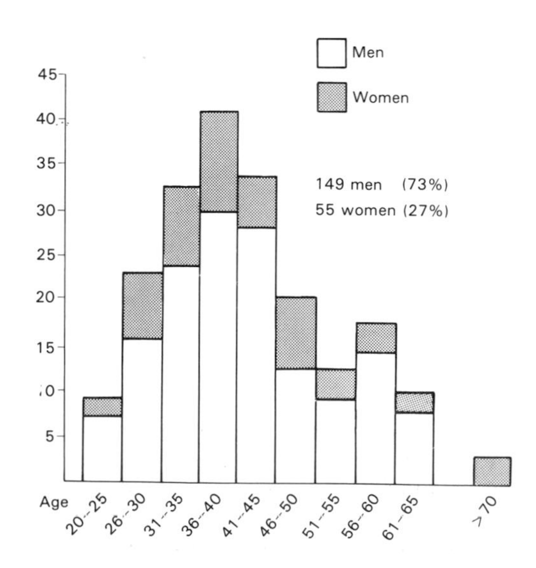

Royal College of General Practitioners: guidelines (units per week)

Low	Women <15	Men <21
Medium	Women 15–35	Men 21–50
High	Women >35	Men >50

Some 27% of men and 11% of women drink above sensible limits and are liable to increasing health risks, while those with the highest intakes will almost certainly have alcohol-related problems. The target set for alcohol in *The Health of the Nation* is a reduction in the proportion of men drinking >21 units to 18% and of women drinking >14 units to 7% by the year 2005.

The justification for asking about alcohol is the problems it can cause. Drinkers are well aware of their problems, but resist making a connection between them and the alcohol. For a long time the family may be caught up in this denial and, indeed, may actively collude with it by tidying up the trail of consequences. The primary care team sees the problems, but may miss the alcohol.

Teenagers with drinking problems are seldom seen in the surgery but may be known to the police for drinking under age or drink-driving offences. Parents may complain that they are out a lot, lethargic, and difficult at home.

Housewives take to drink because they feel lonely or undervalued and this leads to sexual discord, family friction, and even drinking husbands. Women who work outside the home are also at risk, especially in competitive jobs.

The elderly are prone to physical deterioration, intellectual failure, and social isolation. The drinking may be lost in the confusion.

The respected use their status to conceal and their intelligence to rationalise trouble. Regard for them diminishes the critical powers of colleagues, and false loyalties may delay help.

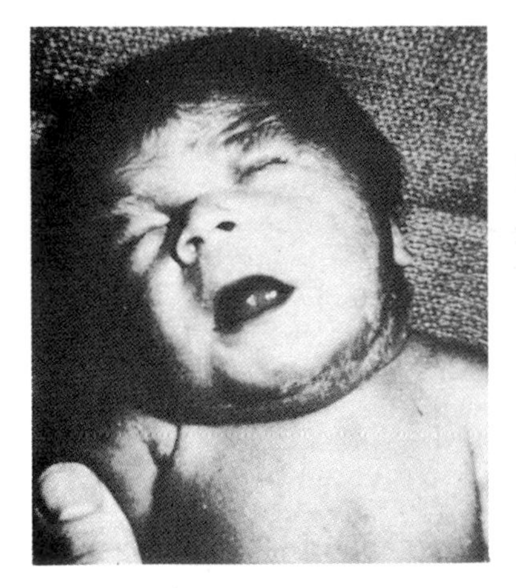

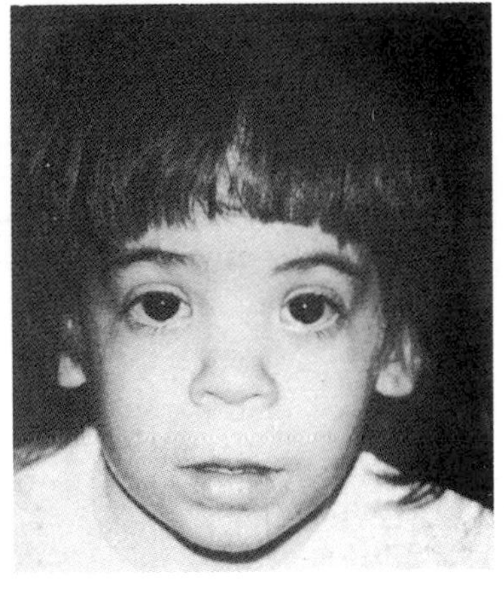

Members of the family are often the presenting sign of a drinking problem, but their prodromal approach is often missed. The general practitioner treats the symptoms without recognising the underlying cause. Non-drinking members of the family suffer too, are patients, and need our care. They are often the best way into a drinking problem, and yield the first rewards for efforts to help.

Children are the most vulnerable members of the family. Infants born to mothers who drink may be damaged. Excessive drinking by the mother in pregnancy is teratogenic and may also cause the fetal alcohol syndrome. Disordered communications cause developmental delay (due to lack of input) or non-accidental injury (violent input). If parents do not respond to simple advice about a child's problems, the general practitioner should ask him- or herself where the block is: alcohol could be the hidden cause.

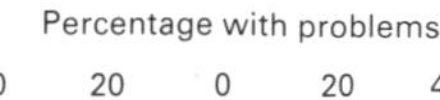

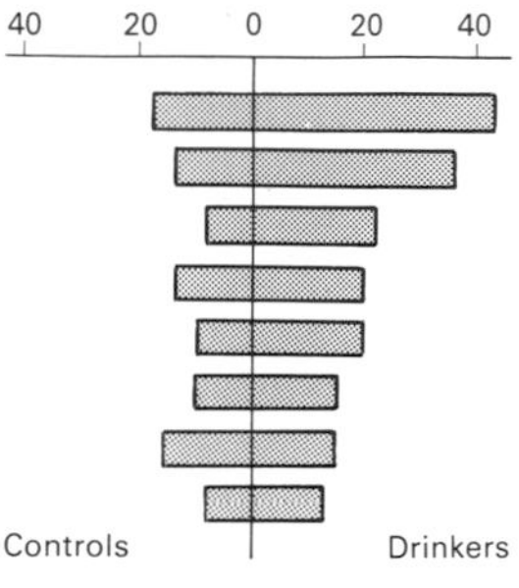

Currently, general practitioners identify only a minority of their patients with drinking problems. The clues are often nonspecific. Doctors and nurses need to think of alcohol every time they meet a clue, and then to check for others in the areas of consumption, physical or psychological or social problems, third-party information, and pathological markers.

Consumption

- Do you drink alcohol?
- What do you drink?
- How much?
- How often?
- Where do you drink?
- Why do you drink?

It has been said that those who reply accurately to being asked how much they drink have no problem. People should be asked if they drink, how often, what, where, and why. As the doctor's acceptance builds confidence, so the amount becomes more discussable. Vagueness, wariness, inconsistencies, evasion or facile assurances need to be addressed, and working back day by day through the past week establishes a retrospective drinking diary. If a patient becomes angered by these questions, it may be because the doctor has inadvertently implied criticism, or because the patient is identifying problems as the cause and not the result of drinking, and is quelling any self-blame by projection onto others.

Problems

Common presenting symptoms

	%
Marital complications	59
Difficulties at work	36
Smelling of alcohol	29
Aggressive behaviour	25
Debts	18
Legal problems	16
Anxiety/depression	13
Gastritis	12
Suicide attempts	5
Others	<4

The physical effects of alcohol misuse are described on page 18 together with the medical conditions for which they are mistaken. In general practice, however, the psychological and social consequences are more important.

Physical examination is seldom helpful apart from the sweating and tremor of early withdrawal, but patients in denial leak a wealth of nonverbal physical signs: in themselves, the evasion or anger already mentioned; in their families and in their homes, the mute testimony of dirt, broken windows, overgrown gardens, and—when concealment is breaking down—empties.

Records

Date	★	CLINICAL NOTES
6.7.79		*Indigestion. Appetite good. Smoking 30/day*
		Advised mag. trisil
2.1.81		*Bruised hand. Tender (R) 5th MP joint. No*
		deformity. Reassured
2.3.81		*Irritable overworking (self-employed now) –*
		not sleeping
		Nitrazepam (20)
12.8.81		*Came late to discuss son's school refusal –*
		slammed out when asked to wait
3.9.81		*More stomach pains – depressed – in laws*
		critical. Smoking ↑ 40. Drinks X 2
		weekly – social
		Hands shaky. Check blood for MCV + γGT
15.9.81		*Last week wife walked out with*
		children. Patient turned car over.
		Breathalyser + Blood alcohol awaited.
		Stands to lose his business (taxi).
		States alcohol no problem – has been
		dry since!
		Resists referral – just wants
		children back.

THIS RECORD IS THE PROPERTY OF THE SECRETARY OF STATE FOR SOCIAL SERVICES

Good notes are a fruitful source of clues that were missed at an earlier stage of the patient's drinking career or of the doctor's awareness. Vague complaints, erratic behaviour, accidental injuries, requests for tranquillisers, and consulting different doctors within the practice are some of these.

No examination of the notes is complete without looking at the notes of the patient's partner and any children. Two-thirds of the commonest presenting symptoms may equally be suffered by other members of the family, who may not themselves be drinking. As with child abuse, the doctor may catch only a fleeting echo of what is happening in the home. Since 67% of incidents of battered women involve alcohol and 70% of abused children have at least one parent who misuses alcohol, perhaps doctors have a duty to put factual cross-references in the notes of other members of the family in order to alert colleagues. If these are on a separate sheet, they do not, as third-party information, contravene the Access to Medical Records Act.

Pathological markers

White blood cell count	7.7×10^9/l
Red blood cell count	4.78×10^{12}/l
Haemoglobin	159 g/l
Packed cell volume	0.467 l
Mean corpuscular volume (MCV)	97.7 fl
Mean corpuscular haemoglobin (MCH)	33.3 pg
Platelet count	295×10^9/l

Creatinine	Uric Acid	Uric Acid
 μmol/l 44–106	0.48 mmol/l M 0.43 F 0.33	 mmol/l
Alk. Phos. 96 Iu/l 40–120 (ADULT)	Bilirubin 13 μmol/l <17	A.S.T. 29 Iu/l <40
C.K. Iu/l M<195 F<170	Amylase Iu/l <220	γGT 78 Iu/l M<50 F<35

Blood alcohol concentrations in drinkers (like blood sugar concentration in diabetic patients) reflect only the immediate situation. As yet we lack a test that reflects alcohol consumption over a period of time with the reliability of a glycated haemoglobin.

In general practice a high mean corpuscular volume (if B12, folate, T4 and thyroid stimulating hormone concentrations are normal) and/or a high γglutamyltransferase (γGT) (if other liver function tests are normal and the patient is not on anticonvulsants) are useful clues. More important is the understanding that people who drink heavily react in one of four ways: *(i)* a rise in mean corpuscular volume, *(ii)* a rise in γglutamyltransferase, *(iii)* a rise in both mean corpuscular volume and γglutamyltransferase, and *(iv)* no rise in either.

Experience in general practice is that the individual characteristic is consistent, and that changes in consumption take some weeks to affect the blood test. Therefore, once a patient is typed, blood tests become, for the first three, both a reliable measure for monitoring future relapses and a useful clue, because many patients have previous routine Coulter Counter or SMAC reports with abnormal results in their notes that were—at the time—ignored.

Communications

> Members of the primary care team have considerable opportunity to identify problem drinkers. The aim must be that not only do they do this but they shall also provide treatment and care.
>
> *Advisory Committee on Alcoholism,* 1978

The practice has a network of communications that can be useful in recognising drinking problems at an early stage. Listening does not compromise confidentiality. Doctors must avoid both the wasteful pursuit of illness-centred diagnoses, and the neglect of any opportunity to pursue their responsibility for the health of those families in their care.

HELP: ADVICE

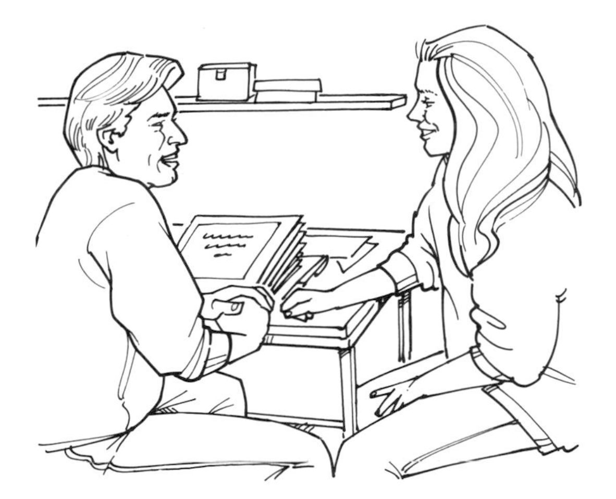

Other articles in this book have shown that alcohol is a health issue and that patients' drinking habits are, like smoking, a matter for clinical inquiry. The doctor has a responsibility to take a drinking history, to advise patients about sensible drinking, and to recognise alcohol-related problems at an early stage.

Many people are sensitive about their drinking, and the offer of help will be more readily accepted if it is given in a spirit of concern for health and the family's wellbeing. It is usually misplaced to be judgmental, and dire warnings are rarely heeded unless they occur in a setting of mutual trust and respect. Once these preconditions exist simple advice from the general practitioner about changing habits is often surprisingly effective.

How to help and how to motivate

BALANCE SHEET

Drinking	Advantages	Disadvantages
Continue	Forget my worries	Lose family
	Escape responsibility	Health deteriorates
		Cost
Reduce	Be like others	I found it hard and
	Appear "normal"	failed last time.
		Wife expects me to
		abstain and doesn't
		believe it possible
Stop	Please wife	What to do with my
	Health improves	time.
	Save money	What to tell my
		drinking friends

Most doctors are pessimistic about being able to help excessive drinkers, yet there is good evidence that as many as two-thirds respond well to treatment. The family doctor is ideally placed to recognise the problem early and intervene.

Motivation is a rather suspect concept. We often blame the patient for lack of motivation when relapse occurs, but, in common with many medical conditions, the treatment of alcohol problems is characterised by relapses and remissions. Relapse is not necessarily the end of the therapeutic road, and the strength of motivation is certainly not constant. A reluctant patient brought by a desperate spouse or coming to avoid dismissal from work can often be converted into taking a personal responsibility for stopping or reducing his or her drinking.

The patient has acquired a drinking habit that is damaging his or her personality, family and social life, or health. Our habits are often hard to change, and the patient will be ambivalent about changing the drinking pattern. This ambivalence can often be addressed directly by asking the patient to draw up a balance sheet of the good and bad consequences of continued drinking.

Armed with such evidence, the patient should set realistic goals for changing his or her lifestyle. It is best to aim for specific short-term goals at first so that the patient gets a sense of achievement by attaining, for instance, three weeks' abstinence or even a party negotiated without disgrace, and then reporting progress. This is often preferable to global but ill-considered promises such as, "I shall never touch another drop." Alcoholics Anonymous embodies the good sense of this approach in its recommendation that the misuser of alcohol should take "only one day at a time".

Changing the lifestyle: impediments and alternatives

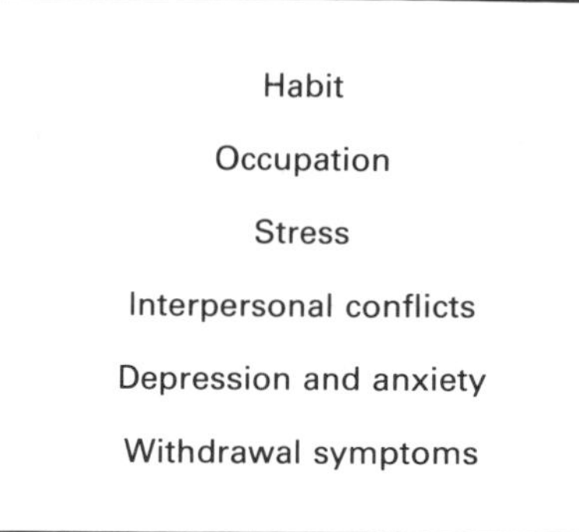
Habit

Occupation

Stress

Interpersonal conflicts

Depression and anxiety

Withdrawal symptoms

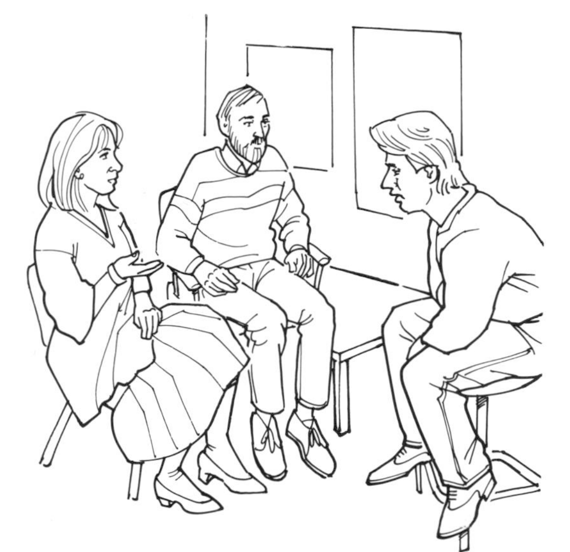

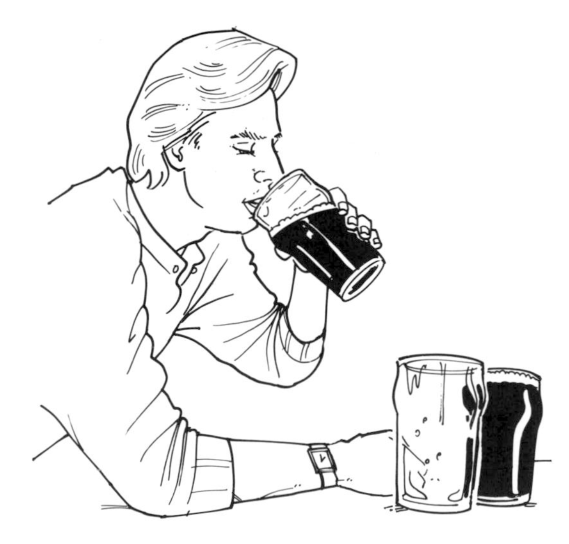

Abstinence

>40 years

Physically addicted

Physical damage

Failed to control drinking

For many problem drinkers drinking has become their predominant interest; to achieve the desired goal they will in time have to make major changes in their way of life. The patient will need help to look at impediments to change and alternatives to drinking.

The impediments will either be evident from the initial balance sheet or become clear as the drinker tries to change his or her habits. Impediments may be, for example, a job where drink is readily available, family stress with which the drinker cannot cope without alcohol, an established neurosis or depression that has been masked by drinking, or the occurrence of withdrawal symptoms when trying to stop drinking. The patient should look out for situations, relationships, and feelings that "trigger" drinking and work out new ways of coping with them. Keeping a diary of drinking occasions is often a helpful way of identifying triggers.

At its simplest patients can be asked to think of activities they enjoy which do not involve drinking. The answer to this question may initially be "none". Alternatives often become clearer if specific attention is paid to past triggers for drinking—for example, the drink at the end of the day may be avoided by going home earlier, the pre-match drink by meeting at the ground itself, and so on. Anxiety as a trigger to drinking may be relieved by appropriate relaxation training. Tranquillisers should not be used for this purpose. Sometimes more elaborate help focused, for example, on tensions in the family may be necessary. The clinician should not discount the more obvious seemingly mechanical and naïve solutions, which often prove surprisingly effective.

Involve the spouse

The spouse is often the prime mover in getting help for the patient. He or she should be actively involved in consultations, partly as an additional source of evidence about the true state of affairs and as an aid to helping the family find a new way of life that does not entail drinking.

The family will have made certain protective adaptations to cope with its drinking members and will need to adjust to the new abstinent personality in its midst. Trust takes time to be re-established and the family will often need support during periods of relapse in which the spouse may feel that all is irretrievably lost. The spouse of an excessive drinker often feels confused, bitter, and devalued, and will welcome the chance of being understood and participating in the process of recovery.

To drink or not to drink

If the drinking is hazardous but hitherto harm-free, the doctor should advise about safe limits for drinking, such as 2 or 3 pints two or three times a week, and clarify the guidelines for sensible drinking, which show that risk of harm begins to increase as consumption rises above 21 units per week for a man and 14 units a week for a woman. The risk of harmful consequences is related to the level of consumption. Drinking should be kept to a minimum during pregnancy (one or two drinks a week), and, of course, when driving or using other complex skills abstinence is the safest policy.

Some drinkers with established problems will return to moderate harm-free drinking, but it is difficult to predict who will succeed where others fail. Present evidence suggest that abstinence remains the safest goal for those who are over 40, are seriously physically addicted, have evidence of physical damage, or have tried controlled drinking treatment without success. For younger people, whose problem drinking has been detected at an early stage and who are not seriously addicted or damaged, modified drinking may be a more acceptable and feasible goal.

Most specialists have probably become less insistent on abstinence as the only goal and are willing to consider modified drinking. This needs to be carefully planned and discussed, and is best preceded by a period of abstinence until evidence of physical harm has disappeared. It is wise to reach agreement about goals with both patients and spouse.

Review

Record exactly what you have drunk on each day last week

	Beers (pints)	Spirits (glasses)	Others including wine (glasses)	Place where consumed
Monday	3			Pub at lunchtime
Tuesday	4	2 whiskies		Pub/friends/evening
Wednesday				
Thursday	8			Evening/friends/payday
Friday	4 (lunchtime) 5 (evening)	2 whiskies		Row with wife
Saturday	2 (lunchtime)		1 bottle wine (dinner)	Home with wife
Sunday	2 (lunchtime)	2 whiskies (evening)		Pub with wife and friends

Whatever the agreed goals, it is essential that the doctor regularly reviews the patient's progress. The most important task at the first interview is to gain the patient's interest in tackling his or her drinking problem and to ensure that he or she returns for the next appointment. At this time the short-term achievements and problems can be reviewed and further goals agreed.

Supportive laboratory tests (γglutamyltransferase, mean corpuscular volume, and breath alcohol) are useful objective means of monitoring progress, and the results and their implications should be discussed with the patient. A diary in which the patient makes a note of any drinks consumed, the time, their quantity, and the occasion is a useful aid to self-audit.

Progress should be reviewed regularly over a year. The first six months of progress often give a good impression of longer term prognosis.

Patients and their families can benefit from reading one of a number of self-help guides to sensible drinking or dealing with problem drinking.

Relapse

What happened?—a behavioural analysis

When?

Where?

Who was there?

How much did I drink?

How often did I drink?

Relapse isn't the end of the road
Set specific short-term goals

Most patients will drink again whatever the original goal of treatment, but this need not be a catastrophic relapse involving the loss of all that has been achieved. It is more profitably viewed as an opportunity for the patient to learn more about his or her nature and the problem. Dealing with and learning from relapses is part of recovery. It needs to be taken seriously by the doctor and patient, and the questions shown opposite need to be honestly asked and answered. Once the anatomy of a relapse is laid bare in this way the patient can recognise strategies for preventing a recurrence. A common cause of relapse is complacency and overconfidence that this problem is in the past and drinking will now be safe.

A closer study of relapses should help patient and doctor to identify triggers to drinking, which may be listed. The family often feels particularly threatened and confused by a relapse and will need extra support at this time. Although there may be setbacks, therapeutic pessimism is misplaced because the long-term prognosis for problem drinkers is surprisingly good.

HELP: RESOURCES

Drugs

Detoxification

- Stop drinking alcohol
- Stay at home for 5 days
- Regular visit from GP or health visitor to maintain physical state, supervise medication and give injections
- Take tranquillisers

The previous article emphasised the importance of gaining the patient's trust and ensuring that regular contact is retained while he or she endeavours to change lifestyle. Drugs have very little place in the long-term management of alcohol problems. They have three principal indications.

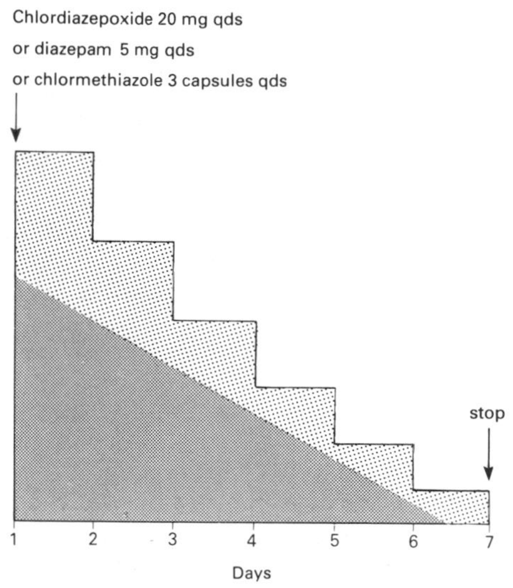

Chlordiazepoxide 20 mg qds
or diazepam 5 mg qds
or chlormethiazole 3 capsules qds

stop

1 2 3 4 5 6 7

Days

Detoxification

Detoxification for the patient who is physically dependent on alcohol may be achieved at home if the patient is willing to stay off work for five days and has a reasonably supportive family. If the patient agrees not to take alcohol, then benzodiazepines may be prescribed in a reducing dose over 5–7 days as shown. Chlormethiazole in a similar regimen may be used, but dependence is a danger if treatment is prolonged, and severe reactions with alcohol may occur. The dose prescribed and the rate of reduction should be related to the clinical state of the patient, but it is not necessary to continue tranquillisers beyond one week. Tranquillisers must not be given on a long-term basis, and the patient should not take them when he or she is drinking. If the patient has a history of withdrawal seizures, detoxification should be started with an increased dose of benzodiazepine.

Oral multivitamin preparations and extra thiamines are often given especially if there is neuropathy, brain damage or obvious poor nutrition.

Alcohol sensitisation

Disulfiram (Antabuse) 200 mg daily is used to sensitise the body to alcohol. The patient who takes this drug and drinks experiences flushing, headache, palpitations, nausea, faintness, and collapse. The reaction may be severe, and patients who have established heart disease should not take the drug. Patients should carry a warning card explaining the dangers of taking alcohol with this drug. Those who can establish the habit of taking disulfiram find it a useful aid to abstinence. It helps if the patient will accept a contract in which he or she agrees to take disulfiram under the supervision of a spouse or some other concerned and responsible person—for instance, an occupational health nurse in an industrial setting. In these circumstances a dose of 400 mg taken on Monday, Wednesday, and Friday is usually sufficient.

Detoxification

Daily check

- Tremor
- Pulse
- Temperature
- Blood pressure
- Level of consciousness
- Orientation
- Dehydration
- Evidence of continued drinking

Psychiatric disorders

Alcohol misuse is sometimes a symptom of an underlying and treatable psychiatric disorder. Depression is a common complaint in excessive drinkers. Occasionally alcohol misuse is symptomatic of an underlying depressive illness, but more often the mood lifts with abstinence. It is wise to postpone consideration of antidepressants until the patient has been abstinent for at least two weeks.

Referral

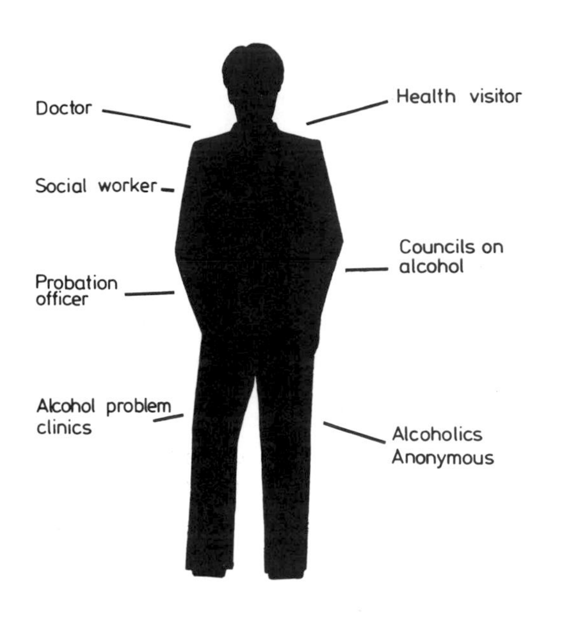

General practitioners may feel that they do not have time to counsel the problem drinker within a busy practice, but this view may not be fully justified. Firstly, the GP already knows a lot about the patient and his or her family and can focus questions and advice quickly. Secondly, the interviews, apart from the assessment with the spouse, which may take 30 minutes, can be conducted in an ordinary surgery. It is probably better to have most interviews short but frequent. Thirdly, the GP has a position of trust and authority, both crucial factors in securing compliance. Finally, the patient and his or her family will attend the surgery anyway—complaining of the symptoms of excessive drinking—so the GP might just as well tackle the underlying cause as patch up the consequences.

As well as the general practitioner, other members of the team, such as health visitors, district nurses, and social workers, are also in a position to take action. The primary care team is thus ideally placed for early intervention, and this alone is often enough. Referral may be necessary, and a variety of agencies and specialist services provide a network of support for people with alcohol problems. The current view is that health districts should support a multidisciplinary community alcohol team, linked with the local hospital and voluntary bodies, and offering counselling and support and a source of information and education about alcohol.

- Severe withdrawal symptoms, particularly fits or delirium tremens—this is a medical emergency
- Lack of supportive environment for withdrawal
- Suspected damage such as decompensated liver disease, peripheral neuropathy, brain damage
- Patient not responding to the approach outlined in this and the previous article
- Presence of underlying neurosis or psychosis
- Very disturbed or unsupportive family
- Need for help in restructuring social activities
- Request for more help with counselling

When to refer

When referral does take place it is important to maintain a relationship with the patient, or he or she may feel like a parcel being passed from one agency to another. It is important to explain the reasons for referral and to check the patient's expectations. Finally, give the patient a further appointment after the consultation with the hospital or other agency so that you can check whether he or she in fact attended (many do not) and discuss views about this new contact.

Alcohol problem clinics (alcohol treatment units)

These are usually associated with psychiatric units; they or district general hospitals have facilities for detoxification. They provide not only specialist consultant services but also training for all types of staff, including volunteers. The services they offer vary considerably, but they generally offer a range of approaches to treatment. As there is no evidence that prolonged inpatient treatment is particularly effective, there is an increasing emphasis on outpatient treatment. Many clinics offer drop-in facilities for patients and relatives and act as day centres. In general the approach has shifted away from being exclusively centred on group psychotherapy and Alcoholics Anonymous to incorporate counselling, marital therapy, training in social skills, and educational approaches.

The simplest advice is to get to know your local unit; the staff will also know about other services in the area.

- Detoxification
- Assessment
- Counselling/psychotherapy
- Social skills training
- Family/marital therapy

Alcoholics Anonymous, Al-Anon, and Al-Ateen

Alcoholics Anonymous (AA) exists throughout Britain; and its membership is growing at the rate of 15% a year. It asks members to acknowledge that they are alcoholic and that abstinence is the only way towards recovery. Some are deterred by its quasi-religious undertones, but there is no requirement to worship or accept religion. Many patients dismiss AA before they have attended often enough to benefit from the fellowship it offers. It is often necessary to shop around before

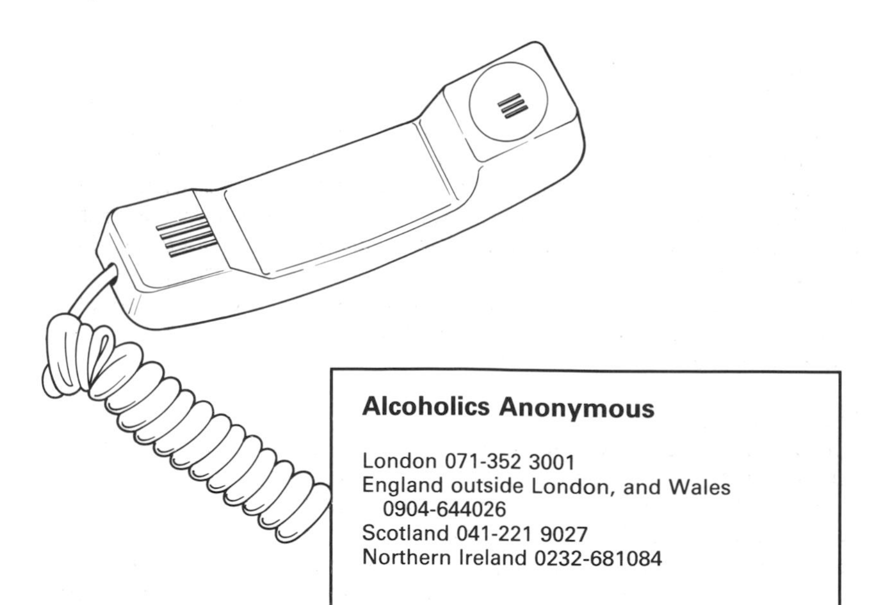

Alcoholics Anonymous

London 071-352 3001
England outside London, and Wales 0904-644026
Scotland 041-221 9027
Northern Ireland 0232-681084

finding a group that suits a particular personality. The GP should get to know a few AA members personally and refer his patients to them. This is much more effective than an open suggestion to attend AA, which many patients are reluctant to do. Some branches operate a 24-hour answering service; the number can be found in the local directory.

Al-Anon and Al-Ateen are organisations that provide support for, respectively, the family and friends and teenage children of excessive drinkers, who can attend in their own right without the patient necessarily belonging to AA. They are especially valuable where heavy drinking has disrupted the family and caused loss of self-esteem and problems over money, care of children, and disposal of property.

Advice about alcohol problems

Many areas have established Councils on Alcohol, voluntary agencies whose responsibilities include coordinating available services and educating and training voluntary counsellors. They also provide free counselling and advice to problem drinkers and their families, and many organise social activities for recovering problem drinkers. Councils will provide information about where to obtain help: some areas have an alcohol information service listed in the telephone directory.

Alcohol Concern has produced a directory of alcohol problem services which cover England and Wales.

Alcohol Concern
275 Grays Inn Road
London WC1X 8QF
Telephone 071 833 3471

Scottish Council on Alcohol
137–145 Sauchiehall Street
Glasgow G2 3EW
Telephone 041 333 9677

Northern Ireland Council on Alcohol
40 Elmwood Avenue
Belfast BT9 6AZ
Telephone 0232 664434

Local advisory services—see telephone directory (under Alcohol)

Self-help publications

Chick, J and Chick, J. *Drinking Problems.* 2nd edn. London: Optima, 1992
Health Education Authority. *That's the Limit: A Guide to Sensible Drinking.* London: 1989
Health Education Board for Scotland. *So You Want to Cut Down Your Drinking.* Edinburgh: 1989
Robertson, I, Heather, N. *Let's Drink to Your Health.* London: British Psychological Society, 1986
Robinson, J. *On the Demon Drink.* London: Methuen, 1989

Alcohol at work

The perspective of these articles has been mainly focused on the family doctor, but hospital doctors and casualty staff are often well placed to offer some of the help and advice described. In the future, occupational health services will probably take on more responsibility for recognising and responding to alcohol problems at work. An increasing number of firms are adopting joint union–management policies to help problem drinkers at work. They guarantee job security to those willing to opt for treatment for their alcohol problem, and this form of "constructive coercion" can be effective.

Patients and their families can benefit from reading one of a number of self-help guides to sensible drinking or dealing with problem drinking.

Many firms have occupational health services that deal confidentially with alcohol problems

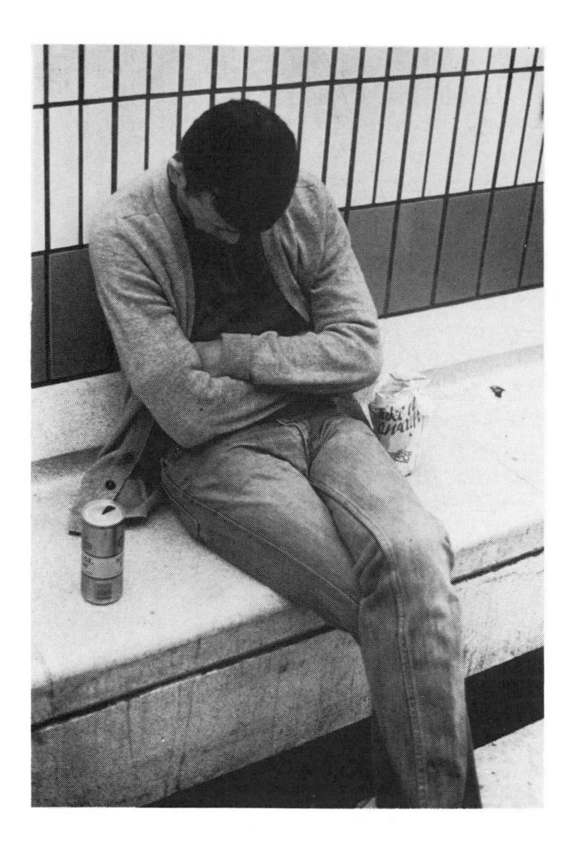

Hostels

Hostels are provided by some local authorities and by voluntary bodies. They cater principally but not exclusively for homeless drinkers and also provide a halfway house for people with alcohol problems discharged from hospital. They have facilities for counselling and rehabilitation. Most require abstinence as a condition of residence. In large cities night shelter accommodation is often provided for vagrant drinkers, who have particular difficulties because they not only need to break away from alcohol but also lack any social framework within which to change. Information about hostels and detoxification centres for drunkenness offenders may be obtained from alcohol advisory services or social work departments.

Probation service

Drunken offenders and people charged with drink-related crimes occupy a great deal of the time of police, courts, and prisons. Drunks arrested and detained in police custody are normally brought before the magistrates the next day; few are referred to the probation service unless they are already under supervision. About a quarter of the clients of the probation service have alcohol problems, and the majority of these people are aged 21–30.

The Probation Service and Social Work have contributed to a number of initiatives in helping individuals where there is a clear link between alcohol misuse and crime. These include educational programmes for drink-driving offenders and young offenders. Some of these benefit if their probation order can be less closely linked to a treatment programme.

Bodies concerned with alcohol

- Alcohol Concern, 275 Grays Inn Road, London WC1X 8QF.
  Tel. 071-833 3471
- Health Education Authority, Hamilton House, Mabledon Place, London WC1H 9TX.
  Tel. 071-383 3833
- Institute of Alcohol Studies, 12 Caxton Street, London SW1H 0QS.
  Tel. 071-222 4001
- Medical Council on Alcoholism, 1 St Andrews Place, London NW1 4LB.
  Tel. 071-487 4445

Sources

Anderson, P. *Management of Drinking Problems.* Euro Series 32. Copenhagen: WHO, 1990

Faculty of Public Health Medicine. *Alcohol and the Public Health.* London: Macmillan, 1991

Heather, N and Robertson, I. *Problem Drinking.* Oxford: OUP, 1985

Royal College of General Practitioners. *Alcohol—a balanced view.* London: RCGP, 1986

Royal College of Physicians. *A Great and Growing Evil: the Medical Consequences of Alcohol Abuse.* London: Tavistock Publications, 1987

Royal College of Psychiatrists. *Alcohol—Our Favourite Drug.* Tavistock Publications, 1986

ACKNOWLEDGEMENTS

The following illustrations are adapted or reproduced by kind permission of the publishers and organisations cited:

p. 1 bottom: reproduced from Office of Health Economics, *Alcohol: Reducing the Harm*, London, 1981; p. 2 bottom: chart adapted from C S Mellor, *BMJ* 1970;**iii**:703; p. 7 top: graph reproduced from Kemm, *Alcohol and Public Health*, Macmillan, 1991; p. 7 bottom: Ledermann curves adapted from an article by Dr J de Lint in *B J Addict* 1975;**70**:3–13; p. 8 top: graph adapted from an article by David Young in *Times* 14 July 1992; p. 10 top: graph reproduced from Office of Health Economics, *Alcohol: Reducing the Harm*, London, 1981; p. 10 bottom: Scope Communications Management; p. 11 bottom: diagram of ethanol metabolism adapted from an article by C S Lieber, *N Engl J Med* 1978;**298**:356; p. 12 middle: graph adapted from Transport and Road Research Laboratory. *The Facts about Drinking and Driving*, Crowthorne, Berkshire, 1983; p. 13 bottom: IBM UK Ltd; p. 14 top left: Brief MAST reproduced from A D Pokorny, B A Miller, H B Kaplan, *Am J Psychiatry* 1972;**129**:342–5; p. 14 top right: "Cage" questions reproduced from D Mayfield, G McLeod, P Hall. *Am J Psychiatry* 1974;**131**:1121–3; p. 15: Lion Laboratories plc, Barry, Wales, UK; p. 16: diagrams of γ-glutamyltransferase and mean corpuscular volume adapted from an article by J Chick, N Kreitman, M Plat, *Lancet* 1981;**i**:249–51, and diagrams of urate and trigylcerides adapted from an article by J B Whitfield, W J Hensly, D Bryden, H Gallagher, *Ann Clin Biochem* 1978;**15**:297–302; p. 21 top: photographs of fetal alcohol syndrome from an article by Sterling K Clarren, *JAMA* 1981;**245**:2436–9; p. 21 bottom: adapted from an article by I C Buchan and others, *J R Coll Gen Pract* 1981;**31**:151–3; p. 29: photograph by Sally and Richard Greenhill.

INDEX

Index